Review Questions and Explanations in
Computed Tomography

Review Questions and Explanations in
Computed Tomography

Lois E. Romans, R.T.(R)(CT)

CT Technologist
Botsford General Hospital
Farmington Hills, Michigan
President
Enterprises for Continuing Education, Inc.
Brighton, Michigan

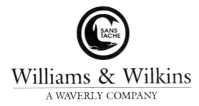

Williams & Wilkins
A WAVERLY COMPANY

BALTIMORE • PHILADELPHIA • LONDON • PARIS • BANGKOK
BUENOS AIRES • HONG KONG • MUNICH • SYDNEY • TOKYO • WROCLAW

1996

Editor: Elizabeth A. Nieginski
Managing Editor: Amy G. Dinkel
Production Coordinator: Danielle Santucci
Copy Editor: Joan A. Coper
Designer: Cathy Cotter
Illustrator: Patricia MacAllen
Typesetting: Maryland Composition
Printer: Port City Press
Binder: Port City Press

Printed in the United States of America

Library of Congress Cataloging in Publication Data

Romans, Lois E.
    Review questions and explanations in computed tomography / Lois E.
Romans.
        p.   cm.
    Companion v. to: Introduction to computed tomography / Lois E.
Romans. c1995.
    Includes bibliographical references and index.
    ISBN 0-683-07330-3
    1. Tomography—Examinations, questions, etc.   I. Romans, Lois E.
Introduction to computed tomography.   II. Title.
    [DNLM: 1. Tomography, X-Ray Computed—examination questions.
2. Anatomy—examination questions.   WN 18.2 R759r 1996]
IN PROCESS
616.07′572—dc20
DNLM/DLC
for Library of Congress   96-1773
                                                                              CIP

*The Publishers have made every effort to trace the copyright holders for borrowed material.
If they have inadvertently overlooked any, they will be pleased to make the necessary
arrangements at the first opportunity.*

                                                    96 97 98 99
                                                    1 2 3 4 5 6 7 8 9 10

Reprint of chapters may be purchased from Williams & Wilkins in quantities of 100 or more. Call Isabella Wise in the Special Sales Department, (800) 358-3583.

Dedication

"It is the supreme art of the teacher to awaken joy in creative expression and knowledge."

Albert Einstein

To my parents, Charles and Rosalie Nastwold, who have the rare ability to awaken the joy of creative expression and knowledge in their children.

Contents

Foreword

Over the years, CT knowledge for technologists has evolved with an emphasis on practical, clinical training and an amazing lack of formal, classroom instruction. This chain of events has produced many technologists who perform adequate, or even excellent, computed tomographic studies. Unfortunately, these operators lack the background information that underlies the reason an exam is performed in a specified way. In effect, technologists have learned how to operate their CT system, but have failed to understand how their CT system operates.

While this type of training definitely works for the short term, that is, it gets the technologist through the daily backlog of patients waiting for scan procedures, it most definitely has drawbacks. Without an understanding of *why* we do what we do, how can we know how other parameters will be affected when one component changes? For example, without an understanding of how contrast media distributes in and is eliminated from the body, how can we know if an adjustment is necessary when scan time is decreased, as is the case of spiral scanning?

Rapidly evolving CT technology demands that the technologist have a good grasp of not only the *how* of specific CT procedures, but also the *why*. While this is an important point, another, perhaps more personally motivating reason for deepening a technologist's CT knowledge, has recently come to pass. That is, the newly implemented advanced certification examinations in computed tomography.

With these new examinations, technologists have found themselves in the unenviable position of being tested on material they were never formally taught. Compounding the difficulty is that comprehensive texts in computed tomography simply do not exist. Much of the material that does exist is not appropriately geared toward technologists. Many textbooks cover anatomy with the comprehensiveness necessary for a radiologist, while ignoring basic operational factors that are essential for the operator.

My intent in writing this book is to serve three main purposes. One is to allow the readers to evaluate their current level of CT understanding and assess possible weak areas for further study. Second, I give brief explanations so that the technologist may bring to the surface knowledge that he or she may have known cognitively. The answers are purposefully brief, although I have included references in the event the reader wishes to pursue a more in-depth study of specific topics. The final goal in writing a question and answer book is to refamiliarize the reader with the process of taking multiple-choice examinations. Often test-taking skills can be improved with practice, and too often technologists, with their original board exam many years in the past, have become rusty at such skills.

I have made every effort to include questions from the entire spectrum of computed tomographic procedures. I have placed an emphasis on deductive reasoning, because it is essential that the technologist be aware of how one adjustment may have myriad consequences.

The questions have been roughly broken down into three main types: (1) questions that concern patient care (20%), (2) those that refer to actual imaging procedures, including the identification of cross-sectional anatomy (50%), and (3) those concerning the physical properties in the production of x-ray and the corresponding generation of the computed tomographic image (30%).

Four practice examinations of 150 questions each contain questions from all of the topics. Answers, often including a brief explanation, can be found at the end of each section.

In the identification of cross-sectional anatomic structures the examinee is at a definite disadvantage in that he or she is allowed to view only the slice displayed. Often it is impossible to absolutely identify a given structure without seeing the images that lie superior and inferior to the one displayed. In such cases, multiple-choice answers will not contain the other plausible choices. For example, an orbit image would not give as choices both the ophthalmic artery and the ophthalmic vein, as these are nearly impossible to differentiate from a single cross-sectional image.

Acknowledgments

This book would not have been possible without the help and support of many people. I would like to extend a special thanks to Dr. Andrew Mizzi of Botsford General Hospital for his help with the aspects dealing with cross-sectional anatomy, physiology, and pathology. Jim Tomlinson from Medical Physics Consultants in Ann Arbor, Michigan, was invaluable in editing the questions on physics and radiation dosimetry. I feel incredibly lucky to have found a physicist who is able to explain his specialty in language I can actually understand. Special thanks to Dr. David Wiseley of Botsford Hospital for setting aside appropriate patient studies for inclusion in this text. Thanks to my dear friend, Mary McGrath, for keeping my three daughters happy and healthy while mommy worked on her book. And finally, I do not have the words to express the gratitude I feel to my husband Ken Romans, RN, for his support, patience, love, and understanding. Not only did he edit the questions concerning patient care, but at least as important, he did the laundry!

Exam 1

Questions

1. Identify the structure indicated by arrow #1 in Figure 1–1.

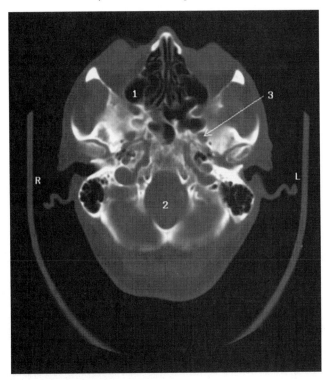

    a. maxillary sinus
    b. ethmoid sinus
    c. sphenoid sinus
    d. roof of orbit

2. Identify the structure indicated by arrow #2 in Figure 1–1.

    a. cerebellar vermis
    b. suprasellar cistern
    c. pons
    d. medulla oblongata

3. Identify the structure indicated by arrow #3 in Figure 1–1.

    a. internal carotid canal
    b. foramen of Magendie
    c. foramen ovale
    d. foramen lacerum

4. Where is the cerebrospinal fluid produced?

    a. choroid plexus
    b. hypothalamus
    c. pons
    d. caudate nucleus

5. Which of the following may be necessary to evaluate suspected rectosigmoid pathology?

   a. A rapid intravenous bolus injection (5 ml/sec or higher) of iodinated contrast media is administered.
   b. 150 to 200 ml of a dilute water-soluble agent is administered by enema.
   c. The pelvis is scanned twice, before and after the administration of an intravenous contrast agent.
   d. The patient should drink 100 ml of oral contrast before scanning; then the patient is scanned in a left decubitus position.

6. Which of the following is appropriate for a computed tomography (CT) study that is performed to rule out an acoustic neuroma?

   a. 8-mm contiguous slices, bone algorithm, filmed at two separate window settings
   b. 5-mm slice thickness with a 4-mm table increment, "soft" (i.e., low- contrast) algorithm, filmed with a narrow window setting
   c. 5-mm contiguous slices, without intravenous contrast, filmed with a narrow window setting
   d. 1.5-mm contiguous slices, standard algorithm initially, retrospectively reconstructed in a bone (i.e., high-contrast) algorithm, filmed at two separate window settings

7. In scanning the posterior fossa in the axial plane, why might an extreme cephalad gantry angle be used?

   a. to avoid dental fillings
   b. to reduce beam-hardening artifacts
   c. to visualize the flow of contrast through the choroid plexus
   d. to visualize the paranasal sinuses

8. The accumulation of serous fluid in the peritoneal cavity is referred to as

   a. asepsis
   b. ascites
   c. flora
   d. aquiparous

9. During a CT examination of the orbit, the patient is asked to fix his eyes on an object. This is done to

   a. reduce radiation exposure to the lens of the eye
   b. help position the patient in the center of the gantry
   c. reduce artifacts
   d. prevent injury to the eye from the laser light used for localization

10. Identify the structure indicated by arrow #1 in Figure 1–2.

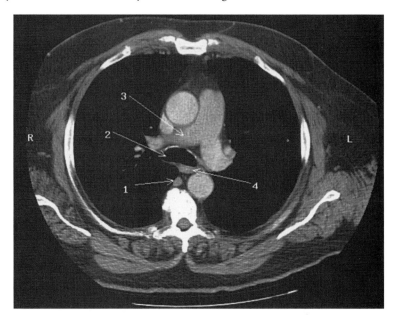

   a. esophagus
   b. vena cava
   c. portal vein
   d. azygos vein

11. Identify the structure indicated by arrow #2 in Figure 1–2.

   a. right main stem bronchus
   b. esophagus
   c. trachea
   d. right middle lobe bronchus

12. Identify the structure indicated by arrow #3 in Figure 1–2.

   a. left atrium
   b. right pulmonary artery
   c. superior vena cava
   d. right brachiocephalic vein

13. Identify the structure indicated by arrow #4 in Figure 1–2.

   a. azygos vein
   b. lymph node
   c. inferior vena cava
   d. esophagus

14. A local or generalized condition in which the body tissues contain an excessive amount of tissue fluid is called

   a. athymia
   b. edema
   c. pericardial effusion
   d. goiter

15. Which of the following is true concerning a routine neck scanning protocol?

    a. Intravenous iodinated contrast media is not necessary in most cases.
    b. Scanning begins near the base of the tongue and ends at the lung apices.
    c. Spiral scanning is not recommended.
    d. A high-contrast, or bone, algorithm should be used.

16. Interstitial disease or subtle air space consolidation is an indication for

    a. CT angiography
    b. multiplanar reformations
    c. aortic dissection protocol
    d. high-resolution chest CT

17. When slice spacing and thickness are equal, images are typically referred to as

    a. spiral
    b. contiguous
    c. continuous
    d. adjacent

18. What type of film is the most common for recording CT images?

    a. single emulsion
    b. double emulsion
    c. cellulose nitrate
    d. rare earth

19. Identify the structure indicated by arrow #1 in Figure 1–3.

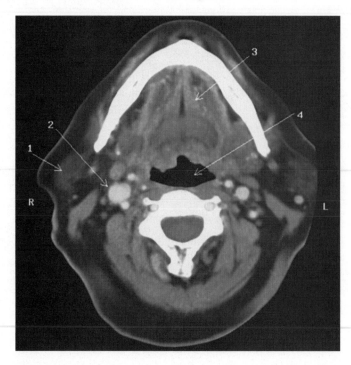

    a. trapezius muscle
    b. external carotid artery
    c. submandibular gland
    d. anterior scalene muscle

20. Identify the structure indicated by arrow #2 in Figure 1–3.

    a. internal carotid artery
    b. internal jugular vein
    c. external carotid artery
    d. vertebral artery

21. Identify the structure indicated by arrow #3 in Figure 1–3.

    a. tongue
    b. epiglottis
    c. strap muscle
    d. pre-epiglottic fat

22. Identify the structure indicated by arrow #4 in Figure 1–3.

    a. vallecula
    b. pyriform sinus
    c. oropharynx
    d. laryngeal vestibule

23. A biphasic injection technique is most often used with which type of CT system?

    a. spiral scanners
    b. fourth-generation systems
    c. electron-beam systems
    d. older, slower scanners

24. It is imperative that all scans be completed before the equilibrium phase of contrast enhancement in studies of the

    a. brain
    b. urinary tract
    c. liver
    d. postsurgical lumbar disk

25. Which of the following structures is also known as the antrum of Highmore?

    a. the posterior horn of the lateral ventricle
    b. putamen
    c. maxillary sinus
    d. internal carotid artery canal

26. When CT is used to evaluate urinary tract calculi, scans should be performed

    a. beginning 90 seconds after the bolus injection of iodinated contrast medium
    b. without intravenous contrast material
    c. with the use of low-osmolality contrast material only
    d. using an iodinated contrast material with a low atomic number

27. One of the abnormalities seen in Figure 1–4 is

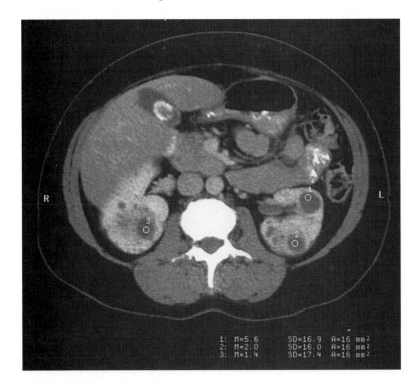

a. kidney stone
b. ascites
c. gallstone
d. aortic dissection

28. A differential diagnosis for Figure 1–4 might be

a. renal papillary necrosis versus renal obstruction
b. polycystic kidney versus multiple single cysts
c. renal carcinoma versus epithelial carcinoma
d. glioma versus islet cell tumor

29. The openings in the roof of the fourth ventricle are the

a. foramen of Monro and foramen rotundum
b. foramen of Magendie and foramen of Luschka
c. foramen ovale and foramen lacerum
d. interventricular foramen and obturator foramen

30. In a CT study, what effects result from a milliampere-second (mAs) setting that is too low?

    1. lower radiation dose to the patient
    2. loss of low-contrast resolution in the image
    3. increased noise in the image
    4. reduced detector efficiency

    a. 1 only
    b. 1 and 3
    c. 1, 2, and 3
    d. 1, 2, 3, and 4

31. What does selecting a small filament size accomplish?

    a. reduces radiation exposure to the patient
    b. concentrates the focal spot
    c. produces a thinner slice
    d. decreases pixel size

32. An adequate CT image is acquired using a scan time of 1 second and 300 milliamperes (mA). Which of the following is likely to result if the technique is changed to a 3-second scan time and 100 mA?

    a. increased tube heat
    b. increased motion artifacts
    c. increased beam hardening
    d. increased image noise

33. In general, which of the following is true of a decrease in slice thickness?

    a. Volume averaging is increased.
    b. mAs can be reduced.
    c. A sharper image is produced.
    d. Voxel size is increased.

34. In Figure 1–5 identify the structure indicated by arrow #1.

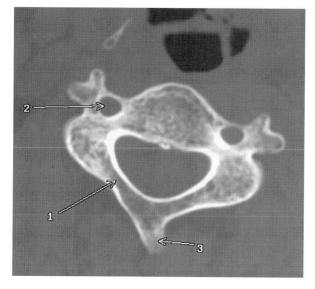

    a. lamina
    b. pedicle
    c. superior articular process
    d. posterior arch (C1)

35. In Figure 1–5 identify the structure indicated by arrow #2.

 a. foramen ovale
 b. foramen rotundum
 c. foramen transversarium
 d. Weitbrecht foramen

36. In Figure 1–5 identify the structure indicated by arrow #3.

 a. transverse process
 b. posterior arch (C1)
 c. spinous process
 d. lamina

37. Figure 1–5 is taken at which level of the spine?

 a. cervical
 b. thoracic
 c. lumbar
 d. sacral

38. Scanning to the adrenal glands in a CT study of the thorax is often performed because

 a. it ensures that the technologist has scanned the entire lung field
 b. kidney function can be assessed
 c. lymph nodes are often visible adjacent to the adrenal glands
 d. lung cancer may occasionally metastasize to the adrenal glands

39. What is the outer portion of the adrenal gland called?

 a. cortex
 b. medulla
 c. omentum
 d. calyx

40. In a spiral scan of the abdomen, the following parameters have been selected: slice thickness = 10 mm, pitch = 1, mA = 250. In this CT system each 360° rotation of the gantry is completed in 1 second. To cover the entire length of the abdomen, a 30-second spiral acquisition is required. However, tube cooling limitations prevent these options. Which of the following options could be substituted?

 a. decrease slice thickness to 5 mm, increase pitch to 2
 b. decrease total acquisition time to 20 seconds, increase pitch to 1.5
 c. decrease slice thickness to 7 mm, decrease mA to 200
 d. increase total acquisition time to 40 seconds, decrease mA to 200

41. A region of interest is measured, and the resultant measurement is 2 Hounsfield units (HU), with a standard deviation of 0. It can be surmised that

 a. all of the pixels within the region have identical values
 b. the area is composed of a variety of different tissue types
 c. the area is likely a calcified nodule
 d. the patient is obese

42. For a CT study of the abdomen, a bolus of 150 ml of contrast is given using a mechanical flow-control injector at a rate of 2 ml/sec. Spiral scanning is begun at 60 seconds after the start of the injection. The liver is seen in which phase of enhancement?

 a. equilibrium phase
 b. nonequilibrium phase
 c. isodensity phase
 d. equalized phase

43. In a lumbar spine scan, which technique helps to differentiate between postsurgical scar tissue and disk disease?

    a. three-dimensional reformations
    b. using a high-contrast, or bone, algorithm and narrow slice thickness
    c. displaying the image with a very wide window width
    d. scanning the spine first without intravenous contrast enhancement and then scanning the surgical area after the administration of an iodinated contrast medium

44. In Figure 1–6 identify the structure indicated by arrow **#**1.

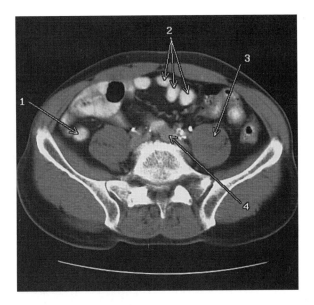

    a. right ureter
    b. ascending colon
    c. descending colon
    d. sigmoid colon

45. In Figure 1–6 identify the structure indicated by arrow **#**2.

    a. hepatic flexure
    b. rectus muscle
    c. transverse colon
    d. sigmoid colon

46. In Figure 1–6 identify the structure indicated by arrow **#**3.

    a. descending colon
    b. mesentery fat
    c. iliacus muscle
    d. greater psoas muscle

47. In Figure 1–6 identify the structure indicated by arrow #4.

    a. left common iliac vein
    b. sigmoid colon
    c. top of bladder
    d. lumbar plexus

48. What can be expected when increasing the pitch in a spiral study from 1:1 to 2:1?

    a. Effective slice thickness is wider than that selected by the collimator opening.
    b. The dose of iodinated contrast medium necessary to perform the scan is increased.
    c. The area of anatomy covered decreases.
    d. The spatial resolution in images increases.

49. In Figure 1–7 identify the structure indicated by arrow #1.

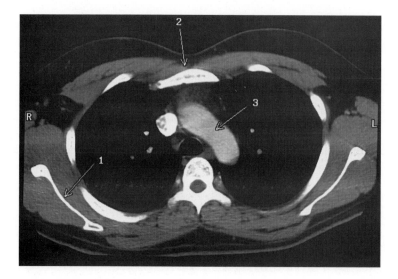

    a. posterior aspect of the third rib
    b. deltoid muscle
    c. scapula
    d. intercostal cartilage

50. In Figure 1–7 identify the structure indicated by arrow #2.

    a. sternum
    b. anterior aspect of the third rib
    c. thyroid cartilage
    d. clavicle

51. In Figure 1–7 identify the structure indicated by arrow #3.

    a. pulmonary artery
    b. right ventricle
    c. left brachiocephalic vein
    d. aortic arch

52. Which of the following is true of three-dimensional reformations of blood vessels?

    a. mAs must be increased by a minimum of 50%.
    b. Thinner slices produce superior three-dimensional models.
    c. Relatively low injection rates (less than 0.8 ml/sec) are used.
    d. Three-dimensional images cannot be created from data acquired in a spiral mode.

53. As a general rule, this is set at a point that has roughly the same value as the average attenuation number of the tissue of interest. What is it?

    a. the x axis in a histogram
    b. standard deviation
    c. sampling rate
    d. window level

54. When performing an abdominal examination on a patient with a history of congestive heart failure, what special action should be taken?

    a. There should be a longer delay between the start of the injection of intravenous contrast material and the start of scanning.
    b. The patient should be pretreated with prednisone.
    c. The patient should be given oxygen.
    d. A thinner slice should be used through the adrenal glands.

55. The trachea bifurcates at the level of

    a. C6–C7
    b. T4–T5
    c. T7–T8
    d. T10–T11

56. What are the names of the two structures located on either side of the sella turcica?

    a. left and right ophthalmic veins
    b. left and right cavernous sinuses
    c. internal and external carotid arteries
    d. inferior and superior orbital fissures

57. Identify the structure indicated by arrow #1 in Figure 1–8.

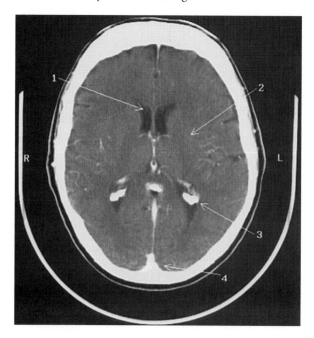

   a. anterior horn of the lateral ventricle
   b. anterior lobe of the internal capsule
   c. third ventricle
   d. habenular commissure

58. Identify the structure indicated by arrow #2 in Figure 1–8.

   a. hypothalamus
   b. putamen
   c. temporal lobe
   d. pons

59. Identify the structure indicated by arrow #3 in Figure 1–8.

   a. pineal gland
   b. posterior cerebral artery
   c. choroid plexus
   d. tentorium cerebelli

60. Identify the structure indicated by arrow #4 in Figure 1–8.

   a. falx cerebri
   b. vein of Galen
   c. cerebellar vermis
   d. superior sagittal sinus

61. Which of the following results from an excess of bilirubin in the blood?

   a. pancreatitis
   b. hemolytic anemia
   c. hemodiastase
   d. jaundice

62. A localized collection of pus in any part of the body that is the result of disintegration or displacement of tissue may be called an

    a. infiltration
    b. apical infection
    c. abscess
    d. inflammation

63. In Figure 1–9 identify the structure indicated by arrow #1.

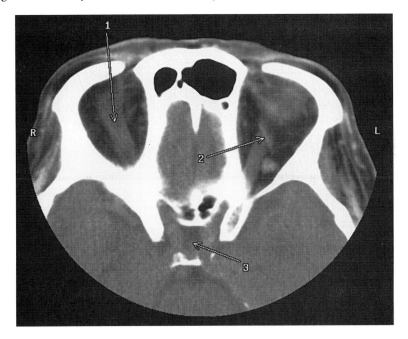

    a. superior rectus muscle
    b. inferior rectus muscle
    c. superior cerebral artery
    d. optic nerve

64. In Figure 1–9 identify the structure indicated by arrow #2.

    a. trigeminal nerve
    b. straight gyrus
    c. ophthalmic vein
    d. basilar artery

65. In Figure 1–9 identify the structure indicated by arrow #3.

    a. prepontine cistern
    b. dorsum sellae
    c. middle cerebellar peduncle
    d. pituitary gland

66. Which of the following is true of nonionic, low-osmolality contrast material?

    a. It is not recommended for spiral studies.

    b. In cases of extravasation, it is less injurious to soft tissue.

    c. It results in a significant difference in relative enhancement of the liver as compared with the ionic type.

    d. Dose can be reduced by 33% when using nonionic contrast, rather than the ionic type.

67. Which specialist is most often involved when performing a stereotactic CT study?

    a. urologist

    b. cardiologist

    c. neurosurgeon

    d. orthopedic surgeon

68. When compared with optical disks, what is an advantage of digital audiotape (DAT) for data storage?

    a. faster image retrieval

    b. superior image quality

    c. less expense

    d. fewer malfunctions

69. The perirenal fascia is also called

    a. Gerota fascia

    b. the cervical fascia

    c. plantar fascia

    d. Cloquet fascia

70. Carbon dioxide has been used in CT studies of the

    a. brain, to counteract seizures associated with iodinated contrast material

    b. spinal canal, to better visualize a herniated disk

    c. bladder, for assessment of intravesicular tumors

    d. orbit, to visualize retinal detachment

71. The area being measured in Figure 1–10 is

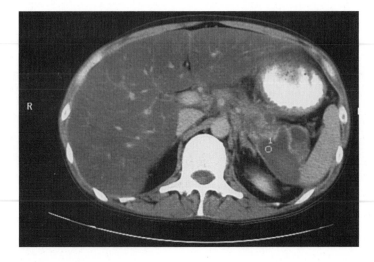

    a. pancreatic pseudocyst

    b. renal cyst

    c. peritoneal blood from a ruptured spleen

    d. adrenal malignancy

72. One of the abnormalities seen in Figure 1–10 is

    a. calcifications within the spleen
    b. ascites
    c. fatty infiltrate of the liver
    d. aortic sclerosis

73. Which of the following is *not* considered a medical asepsis technique?

    a. covering your mouth when you sneeze or cough
    b. autoclaving
    c. hand washing
    d. body substance precautions

74. What is the most common complication from CT-guided needle biopsy?

    a. pneumothorax
    b. peritonitis
    c. bleeding
    d. renal failure

75. When reading a patient's medical chart the abbreviation NPO means

    a. three times per day
    b. nothing by mouth
    c. without fever
    d. as needed

76. Contrast reactions that last briefly and cause symptoms such as nausea, vomiting, itching, sweating, and urticaria are generally classified as

    a. minor reactions
    b. moderate reactions
    c. major reactions
    d. histamine reactions

77. Which units are used to report a partial thromboplastin time (PTT)?

    a. cubic millimeters (mm^3)
    b. seconds
    c. minutes
    d. hours

78. Extensive studies have shown that administration of intravascular iodinated contrast material to pregnant women may result in

    a. a substantially increased risk of miscarriage
    b. an increased rate of birth defects, particularly those relating to the urinary tract
    c. higher than normal birth weights in babies exposed in utero
    d. no impaired fertility or harm to the fetus

79. A pulse that is more rapid than normal is called

    a. bradycardia
    b. hypercardia
    c. tachycardia
    d. cardiorrhexis

80. How should oxygen be administered to patients with pulmonary emphysema or chronic obstructive pulmonary disease (COPD)?

    a. Oxygen should *not* be administered to these patients.
    b. Oxygen should only be given with a written order from the patient's attending physician.
    c. These patients require a high flow rate (6–10 L/min).
    d. These patients require a slow flow rate (2–3 L/min).

81. The systolic figure in a blood pressure recording is a measure of

    a. the pumping action of the heart muscle
    b. the relaxation phase of the heart
    c. the pulse pressure
    d. the amount of blood pumped out of the heart

82. Which of the following describes the system known as body substance precautions?

    a. identification of high-risk patients to enable health care workers to take added precautions
    b. complete removal of all organisms and their spores from all clinical areas
    c. classification of certain body substances, such as blood, as high risk and using gloves when dealing with these substances
    d. use of barriers for all contact with all body substances

83. All of the following are considered standard principles regarding surgical asepsis EXCEPT

    a. never reach across a sterile field
    b. a sterile tray must be used within two hours of being opened
    c. do not pass between the physician and the sterile field
    d. never leave a sterile area unattended

84. What are common side effects from adrenergic agents such as epinephrine (Adrenalin)?

    a. nausea, vomiting, or drowsiness
    b. palpitations, tachycardia, skin flushing, or tremors
    c. confusion, disorientation, or slurred speech
    d. dry mouth, leg cramps, photosensitivity, or rash

85. Which of the following medications may be used as a pretreatment for contrast media reactions?

    1. diphenhydramine
    2. prednisone
    3. atropine
    4. ephedrine

    a. 2 only
    b. 1 and 2
    c. 1, 2, and 4
    d. 1, 2, 3, and 4

86. Following the administration of an iodinated contrast medium, a patient exhibits prominent urticaria. This condition is commonly treated with

    a. an H_1 blocker such as diphenhydramine or an H_2 blocker such as cimetidine
    b. corticosteroids
    c. atropine
    d. a vasopressor such as dopamine

87. Why does the administration of iodinated contrast media result in an enhanced image?

    a. Contrast material increases the ability of the enhanced structure to attenuate the x-ray beam.
    b. Contrast material decreases the average photon energy of the x-ray beam; therefore, more photons are absorbed by the patient.
    c. The administration of contrast material results in a smaller pixel, thereby increasing spatial resolution, which results in an enhanced image.
    d. Contrast material alters the atomic number of body tissues, resulting in decreased attenuations by those structures.

88. Of the following diseases, which has an associated increased risk of impaired renal function?

    a. diabetes mellitus
    b. abdominal aortic aneurysm
    c. biliary obstruction
    d. pancreatitis

89. What is affected when the temperature of contrast media is brought from room temperature to body temperature?

    a. viscosity decreases
    b. osmolality decreases
    c. iodine concentration decreases
    d. rate of extravasation into the surrounding soft tissue increases

90. What is the primary route for contrast media excretion?

    a. vicarious excretion
    b. renal clearance
    c. hepatic excretion
    d. hemodynamic excretion

91. Which of the following are identified by the American College of Radiology as factors that increase a patient's risk for developing an adverse reaction to contrast media?

    1. previous reaction to contrast material (except flushing, heat, nausea, and vomiting)
    2. history of asthma
    3. renal or cardiac impairment
    4. sickle-cell anemia

    a. 1 and 3
    b. 1, 3, and 4
    c. 2, 3, and 4
    d. 1, 2, 3, and 4

92. What criterion must be met for radiation dose to be reported as the computed tomography dose index (CTDI)?

    a. Kilovolt-peak (kVp) must be set at 140, and mAs must be set at 300.
    b. Scanner must be of a third-generation design.
    c. Slices must be contiguous.
    d. Average x-ray beam energy must be less than 70 kiloelectron volts (keV).

93. Before leaving the department after a contrast enhanced CT study has been performed, the patient should be given which of the following instructions?

    a. Refrain from operating heavy machinery for at least 4 hours.
    b. Increase fluid intake for the next 12 hours.
    c. Do not have another examination using iodinated contrast material for a minimum of 3 weeks.
    d. Avoid over-the-counter medications (particularly Tagamet and Pepcid) for at least 4 hours.

94. Which is a *true* statement concerning bowel opacification in a CT study of the abdomen/pelvis?

    a. It is universally accepted that the oral contrast dose should be 300 ml of a dilute barium suspension given 2 hours before scanning.
    b. The rectosigmoid colon can only be distinguished by administering a contrast agent by enema.
    c. In general, the greater the volume of oral contrast material, the better the bowel opacification.
    d. Conventional radiography suspensions can be used in CT and are less expensive than the specialized CT suspensions.

95. This laboratory value is a measure of the number of circulating platelets in venous or arterial blood. A low count results in prolonged bleeding time and impaired clot retraction. This laboratory test is commonly called a

    a. platelet count
    b. prothrombin time (PT)
    c. creatinine
    d. white cell count

96. The use of a flow-control pressure injector is recommended for CT studies of the body because

    a. there is a reduced risk of extravasation of the contrast media into the soft tissues
    b. side effects such as heat and nausea are reduced
    c. contrast media dose and timing can be easily regulated and reproduced in subsequent studies
    d. the risk of air embolus is eliminated

97. Which is a *disadvantage* of the hand bolus method of contrast enhancement?

    a. It has slower flow rates than the drip infusion method.
    b. The operator may be exposed to scatter radiation.
    c. It is impossible to reach peak contrast enhancement due to slow flow rates.
    d. Plasma iodine concentration never reaches as high as with the drip infusion method.

98. Which of the following is *true* of an ionic contrast medium?

    a. All ionic contrast media have high osmolality.
    b. Ionic contrast media are typically more expensive than the nonionic types.
    c. The molecules in an ionic contrast solution dissociate to form ions in water.
    d. Ionic contrast agents have fewer particles in solution than nonionic agents.

99. Which are advantages of low-osmolality contrast agents (Omnipaque® or Optiray®)?

    1. Osmolality is identical to body fluids.
    2. There are fewer adverse reactions than from high-osmolality agents.
    3. Fatal reactions are eliminated.
    4. They are less damaging to the soft tissues in cases of extravasation.

    a. 1 and 2
    b. 2 and 4
    c. 1, 2, and 4
    d. 1, 2, 3, and 4

100. A possible complication from the oral administration of a barium sulfate solution is

    a. barium toxicity
    b. dehydration
    c. aspiration pneumonitis
    d. overdose

101. In scanning the abdomen, what can be done if the patient is unable to take fluids by mouth?

    a. The volume of intravenous contrast is increased by 25% to compensate for the lack of an oral contrast medium.
    b. 200 ml of a dilute water-soluble agent is administered by enema.
    c. A nasogastric tube may be inserted for the administration of an oral contrast agent.
    d. A small volume of a dilute water-soluble contrast agent can be administered by an inhaler.

102. When performing a CT study of the abdomen, which of the following is recommended for the intravenous injection of iodinated contrast media?

    a. 1 1/2 inch, 16-gauge needle
    b. 21–23-gauge butterfly needle
    c. 18–20-gauge needle with a flexible plastic cannula
    d. 15 cm, 20–22-gauge Chiba needle

103. When intravenous contrast media are used in pediatric scanning, the usual dose is (60% solution of intravascular contrast media containing approximately 280 mg iodine/ml)

    a. 0.5 ml/kg to a maximum of 1 ml/kg or 25 ml
    b. 1 ml/kg to a maximum of 2 ml/kg or 50 ml
    c. 2 ml/kg to a maximum of 4 ml/kg or 100 ml
    d. 4 ml/kg to a maximum of 8 ml/kg or 150 ml

104. Which is *true* regarding the fetal risk when a pregnant woman is exposed to ionizing radiation?

    a. The risk of congenital abnormalities is significant, even with exposures of less than 1 rad.
    b. The fetus is most vulnerable to radiation-induced congenital abnormalities during the last trimester.
    c. The risk is negligible with an exposure of 10 rads in the second or third trimester of gestation.
    d. The fetal risk depends on the gestation period.

105. Increasing the scan field of view

    a. increases the number of detector cells collecting data
    b. increases the range of HU displayed on the image
    c. decreases the pixel size
    d. decreases the display field of view (zoom, target)

106. A CT slice is taken with the following factors: mA = 300, scan time = 1 second, matrix = 512, kVp = 120, slice thickness = 10 mm. The resulting image is suspected of containing a considerable amount of volume averaging. Which of the above factors is *primarily* responsible?

    a. mA
    b. scan time
    c. matrix
    d. slice thickness

107. A grid formed from columns and rows of pixels is called a

    a. back projection
    b. convolution filter
    c. matrix
    d. histogram

108. When comparing the beam attenuation capacity in metallic objects to that of substances such as fat or air, which is a true statement?

    a. Because they absorb a large percentage of the x-rays that strikes them, metallic objects have greater beam attenuation capacity.
    b. Because metallic objects are represented on film as light shades of gray, they can be said to possess a small beam attenuation capacity.
    c. Metallic objects create very narrow gray scales but have no effect on beam attenuation.
    d. Although metallic objects have a great capacity for beam attenuation, it is not nearly as high as that of either air or fat.

109. What unit quantifies a structure's beam attenuation?

    a. mAs
    b. million heat units (MHU)
    c. line pairs (lp)
    d. HU

110. In what part of the CT system are the components that produce x-rays housed?

    a. the central processing unit (CPU)
    b. the data acquisition system (DAS)
    c. the gantry
    d. the transformer unit

111. The ability of the tube to withstand by-product heat is called

    a. heat capacity
    b. heat dissipation
    c. thermal potential
    d. thermal transference

112. In the production of a CT image, approximately how often are the detector cells sampled?

    a. 1000 times a minute
    b. once a second
    c. 50 times a second
    d. 1000 times a second

113. Which component of the CT system converts the electric signal supplied by the detectors into a digital format?

    a. photodiode
    b. array processor
    c. digital-to-analog converters
    d. analog-to-digital converters

114. Which components are used in the data acquisition phase of image creation?

    a. generator, gantry, patient table
    b. reconstruction processor, display processor, cathode-ray tube (CRT) monitor
    c. analog-to-digital converters, array processor, magnetic optical disk
    d. digital-to-analog converters, array processor, CRT monitor

115. The configuration of the x-ray tube to the detectors determines a scanner's

    a. heat dissipation rate
    b. detector efficiency
    c. generation
    d. speed

116. Which statement is true concerning a fourth-generation design?

    a. All spiral/helical scanners are of the fourth-generation design.
    b. Ring artifacts are more common in fourth-generation systems as compared with the third-generation design.
    c. A lower technique can be used with a fourth-generation system than with a third-generation system (all other factors remaining the same).
    d. Since the fourth-generation design was introduced, third-generation scanners are rapidly becoming obsolete.

117. Which are advantages of filtering the x-ray beam?

    1. Filtering produces a more uniform beam, thereby reducing beam-hardening artifacts.
    2. mA settings can be decreased with a filtered beam, thereby alleviating stress on the x-ray tube.
    3. A filtered beam produces images with substantially less quantum mottle.
    4. Filtering minimizes patient radiation exposure.

    a. 1 and 4
    b. 1, 2, and 4
    c. 2, 3, and 4
    d. 1, 2, 3, and 4

118. Xenon gas and solid-state crystals are

    a. the two most common materials used in an array processor
    b. used together to create the computer chips used by the CPU
    c. materials used to cool the x-ray tube
    d. the two main varieties of detectors currently in use

119. In a CT system, the process of generating x-ray photons results in most of the energy being converted to

    a. light
    b. an electric charge
    c. x-rays
    d. heat

120. All of the thousands of bits of data acquired by the CT system with each scan are called

    a. image data
    b. calibration vectors
    c. raw data
    d. ray sums

121. What is a disadvantage of a small x-ray tube filament?

    a. reduced spatial resolution
    b. reduced detector efficiency
    c. increased penumbra
    d. reduced heat capacity

122. What is the most common reason for using an overscan?

    a. to reduce motion artifacts, particularly in fourth-generation scanners
    b. to increase the total radiation exposure to the patient
    c. to allow more refined calibrations during the scan process
    d. to reduce ring artifacts in third-generation scanners

123. Why is a third-generation system sometimes referred to as a rotate–rotate scanner?

    a. The tube first rotates in one direction, then stops to rotate in the opposite direction.

    b. The tube continues to rotate in the same direction.

    c. The tube and detector rotate in unison, facing opposite one another.

    d. The tube and detector each rotate in the opposite direction.

124. Which of the following statements best summarizes the Nyquist sampling theorem?

    a. Because an object may not lie entirely within a pixel, the pixel should be half the size of the object to increase the likelihood of being resolved.

    b. It offers information on the resolution capability of the scanner as a function of spatial resolution.

    c. It offers a graphical representation of the system's capability of passing information through it to the observer.

    d. It is the process of determining the unknown value of a function between known values of the function.

125. Which of the following statements best describes the contrast–detail response?

    a. It is used to explain the fact that different observers look at the same image and evaluate it differently.

    b. For a given technique, the level of contrast that is visible diminishes as the object size decreases.

    c. Because an object may not lie entirely within a single pixel, pixel size should be no more than half the size of the object.

    d. Resolution decreases as pixel size increases.

126. Which two factors may produce a grainy appearance in the image?

    a. too low mAs setting or low tube output

    b. faulty detector or too few samples

    c. patient not entirely enclosed in scan field or insufficient x-ray beam filtration

    d. angle of x-ray beam varying between two similar views or the x-ray beam composed of different energies

127. Broad streaks in the image, cupping where the periphery of the image is lighter, and vague areas of low density are all manifestations of

    a. quantum mottle

    b. the aliasing effect

    c. air–contrast interface artifacts

    d. beam-hardening artifacts

128. What is the range of pixel values represented on an image where the window width is set at 1600 and the window level is set at −200?

    a. −1800 to 1400

    b. −1000 to 600

    c. 1400 to 1800

    d. −800 to 800

129. Which factors influence the linear attenuation coefficient for a material?

    a. pixel size and scanner generation

    b. scan time and algorithm

    c. nature of the material and photon energy of the beam

    d. mA setting and display field of view

130. On a CT image a structure is measured, and its CT number, or HU, is −90. It is most likely composed of

    a. gray matter

    b. lung

    c. water

    d. fat

131. Which of the following affects the anode heat loading on a CT tube?

    a. slice thickness
    b. algorithm
    c. kVp
    d. display field size

132. The spatial resolution of a scanner worsens if there is a decrease in

    a. focal spot size
    b. slice thickness
    c. matrix size
    d. mA

133. Which of the following reduces scatter radiation?

    a. increasing the slice thickness
    b. increasing the filtration
    c. decreasing the kVp
    d. decreasing the display field size

134. When slice thickness is decreased, which other factor should be adjusted?

    a. A sharper algorithm should be selected.
    b. mAs should be increased.
    c. Scan field size should be decreased.
    d. Display field size should be decreased.

135. In CT, what is a "space charge"?

    a. the charge within the xenon gas detector after it has been struck by an x-ray photon
    b. when the space between detectors becomes ionized
    c. the cloud of electrons that are emitted from a heated filament
    d. the amount of charge an element would have if it were contained within a vacuum

136. What is the approximate pixel size if a 512^2 matrix is used with a 25-cm field of view?

    a. 0.5 mm
    b. 0.5 cm
    c. 2.0 mm
    d. 2.0 cm

137. Which factors may affect the HU assigned to a pixel in a CT image?

    1. structure heterogeneity
    2. tissue density
    3. atomic number of the structure
    4. contrast enhancement of the structure

    a. 1 and 4
    b. 1 and 2
    c. 2 and 3
    d. 1, 2, 3, and 4

138. Decreasing the window width in a CT image decreases

    a. slice thickness
    b. mAs
    c. the appearance of quantum mottle
    d. the anatomic diversity displayed

139. Which of the following statements is true concerning beam-hardening artifacts?

    a. They are affected by x-ray beam filtration.
    b. They increase all CT numbers on the image.
    c. They occur only with third-generation systems.
    d. They cause white rings in the CT image.

140. Of the following factors, which affects the detection of large, low-contrast objects?

    1. window setting
    2. mA
    3. scan time
    4. patient size

    a. 1 only
    b. 4 only
    c. 2 and 3
    d. 1, 2, 3, and 4

141. What is required for a CT system to have a variable kVp output?

    a. two or more focal spot sizes
    b. two or more filaments
    c. a more sophisticated generator
    d. a rotating anode

142. Digitized data from the computer processing unit is converted into shades of gray by the

    a. display processor
    b. array processor
    c. photodiode
    d. DAS

143. A major advantage of spiral scanning over conventional CT is

    a. the center of the reconstructed section can be retrospectively and arbitrarily placed along the z axis
    b. the software that corrects for table motion also eliminates patient motion artifacts such as cardiac pulsations and peristalsis
    c. even with a pitch of one or less, radiation dose is reduced by more than half
    d. slice thickness can be narrowed retrospectively

144. What type of data does archiving devices such as optical disks and magnetic disks store?

    a. raw data
    b. image data
    c. scan data
    d. all data collected from the detectors

145. A phantom is scanned, and the average CT numbers from the resulting image are plotted as a function of the attenuation coefficients of the phantom materials. This is used to demonstrate the system's

    a. linearity
    b. noise
    c. spatial resolution
    d. heat dissipation rate

146. What is necessary to perform a sagittal reformation?

    1. Images must have identical gantry tilts.
    2. Images must have the same display field of view.
    3. Images must be contiguous.
    4. Images must share the same center.

    a. 1 and 3
    b. 2 and 4
    c. 1, 2, and 3
    d. 1, 2, 3, and 4

147. In a three-dimensional reformation, what is it called when a specific bone is isolated for viewing?

    a. disarticulation
    b. disjointing
    c. infraction
    d. transgressing

148. An area is scanned, and it is discovered that vital anatomy has not been included on the image. What is necessary to display the missing anatomy on the image?

    1. The system must have a magnification option.
    2. The original display field size must be smaller than the scan field size.
    3. The raw data must be available.
    4. The image data must be available.

    a. 1 and 2
    b. 2 and 4
    c. 2 and 3
    d. 2, 3, and 4

149. An advantage to spiral scanning over conventional axial scanning is that

    a. spiral images permit a more effective, focused use of contrast media
    b. spiral images provide superior, spatial resolution
    c. slice thickness can be adjusted retrospectively
    d. tube heat loading is reduced because of the shortened exam time

150. If the raw data are used again to create a new image after the initial image has been generated, it is typically referred to as

    a. multiplanar reformation
    b. archiving
    c. retrospective reconstruction
    d. creating a mask

Answers and Explanations

1. **Answer-a**

2. **Answer-d**

3. **Answer-c**

4. **Answer-a.** Cerebrospinal fluid produced in the choroid plexus seeps into the lateral ventricle via a network of capillaries. From there it seeps through an opening called the interventricular foramen (of Monro) into the third ventricle.

5. **Answer-b.** In evaluating the rectosigmoid area, it is helpful for the bowel to be contrast filled. This is sometimes achieved by having the patient drink at least 600 ml of oral contrast at least 6 hours before the examination. Contrast may be given rectally if the oral contrast fails to opacify the rectosigmoid colon. In these cases, 150 to 200 ml of a 1% to 3% water-soluble agent is administered by enema.

6. **Answer-d.** Because very small structures are being evaluated, it is recommended that the thinnest slice available be used for scanning the internal auditory canal. The technique calls for the initial images to be processed with a standard algorithm and filmed with a narrow window setting. The raw data are then used to create images with a high-contrast, or bone, algorithm, and these are filmed using a wide window setting. This is performed to check for any bony deterioration. Magnetic resonance imaging (MRI) is currently the examination of choice for the evaluation of acoustic neuromas.

7. **Answer-b.** This technique is often referred to as reverse angle imaging of the posterior fossa. It is designed to reduce beam-hardening artifacts and thereby improve visualization of the structures of the posterior fossa.

8. **Answer-b**

9. **Answer-c.** Having the patient fix his eyes on an object reduces ocular motion, thereby reducing motion artifacts on the image.

10. **Answer-d**

11. **Answer-a**

12. **Answer-b**

13. **Answer-d**

14. **Answer-b**

15. **Answer-b.** Neck scans are performed with either a standard or soft algorithm. Spiral scanning can be advantageous by allowing all scans to be acquired at peak contrast enhancement and while the patient suspends swallowing. Intravenous contrast media administration is considered essential in computed tomography (CT) studies of the neck.

16. **Answer-d.** A high-resolution chest scanning protocol incorporates very thin slices taken with a spacing of 10 mm or more. These are reconstructed using a high-contrast, or bone, algorithm.

17. **Answer-b.** Slice spacing options in conventional axial scanning are overlapping, gapped, or contiguous. In spiral scanning the slice spacing option is replaced by pitch.

18. **Answer-a.** Single-emulsion film is used in recording CT images. Cellulose nitrate is a material that was used as a base material for x-ray film in the 1920s. Its use was discon-

tinued because it is extremely flammable and several radiology departments burned down because of it. Intensifying screens used in standard radiography use rare earth phosphors.

19. **Answer-c**

20. **Answer-b**

21. **Answer-a**

22. **Answer-c**

23. **Answer-d.** A biphasic technique allows an initial bolus of contrast to reach peak enhancement, followed by a slower second phase that maintains enhancement until the scanner can complete the study.

24. **Answer-c.** If scans are acquired in the equilibrium phase, liver lesions may become isodense and, therefore, indistinguishable.

25. **Answer-c.** The maxillary sinus is the largest of the four paranasal sinuses.

26. **Answer-b.** "Although CT is not the primary diagnostic technique for evaluating urinary tract calculi, when it is employed, it should be performed without intravenous contrast injection, as contrast material obscures the diagnosis in more than 75% of instances."[1]

27. **Answer-c**

28. **Answer-b**

29. **Answer-b.** The foramen of Magendie and foramen of Luschka permit the flow of cerebral spinal fluid into the subarachnoid space.

30. **Answer-c.** In addition to reducing the radiation exposure to the patient, image noise is increased because too few x-ray photons reach the detectors. Whenever noise increases, low-contrast resolution decreases. Detector efficiency is not affected by milliampere-seconds (mAs).

31. **Answer-b.** Concentrating the focal spot improves spatial resolution by reducing blur. Assuming all other factors are kept constant, there will not be a change in slice thickness, radiation dose, or pixel size.

32. **Answer-b.** A longer scan acquisition time allows more opportunities for voluntary and involuntary patient motion.

33. **Answer-c.** When slice thickness is decreased, mAs must be increased to compensate. If this adjustment in mAs is made, a sharper image results from the corresponding decrease in volume averaging. Voxel size is decreased.

34. **Answer-a**

35. **Answer-c**

36. **Answer-c**

37. **Answer-a**

38. **Answer-d.** Often scanning of the thorax is continued past the lung bases to the adrenal glands. This is done because a small percentage of patients with a primary lesion of the lung have metastasis to the adrenal gland. Scanning to the adrenals is typical in patients with a history of cancer. For all other patients, a chest scan is complete when the lung field has been covered.

[1] Moss A, Bush W: Abdomen and pelvis. In *Computed Tomography of the Body, with Magnetic Resonance Imaging*, 2nd ed, vol 3. Edited by Moss A. Philadelphia, WB Saunders, 1992, p 982.

39. **Answer-a.** The outer portion of the adrenal gland is called the cortex, and the inner substance is called the medulla. Although the adrenal cortex and the adrenal medulla are structurally part of one organ, they function as separate endocrine glands.

40. **Answer-b.** By increasing the pitch to 1.5, the total acquisition time can be decreased to 20 seconds and still cover the entire 300 mm of anatomy.

41. **Answer-a.** The measurement of 2 Hounsfield units (HU) is the average of all pixel values within the region of interest. The standard deviation indicates the amount of CT number variance within a region of interest. If the standard deviation is 0, there is no variance; therefore, each of the pixels within the region measures 2 HU.

42. **Answer-b.** The nonequilibrium phase, which follows the bolus phase, is characterized by a difference of 10 to 30 HU between the aorta and the inferior vena cava. The last phase is called the equilibrium phase, which is when contrast is equalized between tissues. In the equilibrium phase, tumors of the liver may become the same density (isodense) as the normal liver tissue and, therefore, be undetectable.

43. **Answer-d**

44. **Answer-b**

45. **Answer-c**

46. **Answer-d**

47. **Answer-a**

48. **Answer-a.** Because of the spiral motion and the process of interpolation applied to the spiral data, the true slice is wider in spiral scanning than in conventional CT for the same chosen slice thickness. This widening is slight when the pitch is kept at 1:1, but effective slice thickness becomes progressively wider as pitch increases. The most profound slice thickness blooming occurs when pitch surpasses 1.5:1.

49. **Answer-c**

50. **Answer-a**

51. **Answer-d**

52. **Answer-b.** CT angiography is typically performed with a slice thickness of 5 mm or less. Injection rate usually ranges from 2 to 3 ml/sec. It is not necessary to increase mAs on the initial scans. Spiral data make excellent three-dimensional reformations because the data can be retrospectively reconstructed with a 50%, or greater, overlap.

53. **Answer-d.** It is customary to set the window level at the same approximate value as the attenuation number of the area of interest (i.e., a common window level for an abdomen study is 50, whereas a brain study often uses a window level of 30).

54. **Answer-a.** Because the heart works less effectively in patients with congestive heart failure, the circulation time is prolonged. As a result, an intravenous contrast agent takes longer to reach the scanned structures.

55. **Answer-b.** The trachea begins at the level of the sixth cervical vertebra and bifurcates near the fourth or fifth thoracic vertebra. The bifurcation of the trachea is referred to as the carina.

56. **Answer-b.** The cavernous sinuses originate anteriorly at the ophthalmic vein and terminate at the petrosal sinuses. They communicate with each other by means of the circular sinus.

57. **Answer-a**

58. **Answer-b**

59. **Answer-c**

60. **Answer-d**

61. **Answer-d.** Jaundice is a condition characterized by the yellowness of the skin, whites of the eyes, and mucous membranes.

62. **Answer-c**

63. **Answer-a**

64. **Answer-c**

65. **Answer-d**

66. **Answer-b.** In studies on laboratory animals, nonionic contrast medium has been shown to be less injurious to cutaneous and subcutaneous tissue than conventional ionic, high-osmolar contrast material.[2]

67. **Answer-c.** The use of a stereotactic device in conjunction with CT imaging can provide essential information for the neurosurgeon. This system can provide exact localization of a specific pathological target.

68. **Answer-c**

69. **Answer-a.** The fascia is a fibrous membrane covering that supports and separates muscles. It also connects the skin with underlying tissue. The fascia can be either superficial or deep. The cervical fascia is located in

the neck; the plantar is in the foot; and Cloquet fascia is in the femur. Gerota fascia and the lateroconal fascia divide the anterior and posterior pararenal compartments.

70. **Answer-c.** Carbon dioxide provides a negative contrast agent when administered by catheter into the bladder. The main advantage of using carbon dioxide over iodinated contrast medium is that the gas does not obscure these tumors, as dense contrast medium may.

71. **Answer-a**

72. **Answer-c**

73. **Answer-b.** Medical asepsis techniques are those that inhibit the growth and spread of disease-causing microorganisms. Autoclaving is a method of sterilization and, as such, eliminates all microorganisms. It is considered a technique of surgical asepsis.

74. **Answer-c.** Although pneumothorax may be the most common complication in biopsy procedures performed in the thorax, overall, the most common complication of all biopsy procedures (including the thorax, abdomen, and pelvis) is bleeding, which occurs in approximately 2% of cases.

75. **Answer-b**

76. **Answer-a.** Reactions are classified into four groups: minor, moderate, major, and fatal. Minor reactions are those that resolve quickly. Generally, no treatment is required.

77. **Answer-b.** The normal range is 24 to 36 seconds.

78. **Answer-d.** Reproduction studies have been performed in rats and rabbits with up to 100 times the recommended human dose. No

2 Cohan RH, Leder RA, Bolick D, et al: Extravascular extravasation of radiographic contrast media. *Investigational Radiology* 25:504–510, 1990.

evidence of impaired fertility or harm to the fetus due to intravascular iodinated contrast media has been demonstrated. However, there are no studies in pregnant women. Because animal reproduction studies are not always predictive of the response in humans, iodinated contrast material should be used during pregnancy only if essential.

79. **Answer-c.** Tachycardia is when the pulse rate is over 100 beats/min. It may result from excitement, exertion, or a damaged heart. Tachycardia may indicate interference with oxygen supply or loss of blood.

80. **Answer-d.** Not all patients with breathing problems require oxygen at a high flow rate. Conditions such as pulmonary emphysema or chronic obstructive pulmonary disease (COPD) necessitate a slow rate of oxygen flow to provide additional oxygen but not depress respirations.

81. **Answer-a.** Blood pressure is often defined as the pressure exerted by the blood on the walls of the vessels. It consists of two numbers, the systolic and diastolic pressures. The systolic pressure indicates the force of the contraction that empties the ventricles to push blood into the aorta.

82. **Answer-d.** Body substance precautions, or universal precautions, is a system based on the use of barriers for every contact with any body substance. It replaces the older system of isolating patients with a particular diagnosed disease. This system is recommended by the Centers for Disease Control, which stress that this approach should be used on *all* contact with *all* body substances of *all* patients at *all* times.

83. **Answer-b.** Once opened, a sterile object must be used immediately because airborne contamination may occur.

84. **Answer-b.** These side effects are usually mild and generally resolve untreated. It is important to recognize these symptoms as side effects of epinephrine and not assume that they are an escalation of the allergic response that they were given to counteract.

85. **Answer-c.** Atropine is not used to premedicate. It is typically administered when a vagal reaction results from the injection of contrast media. Atropine is classified as an anticholinergic; it depresses the parasympathetic nervous system and acts as an antispasmodic of the gastrointestinal tract. In addition to prednisone (a corticosteroid), ephedrine, and diphenhydramine (Benadryl), cimetidine (Tagamet) also has been used in the pretreatment of contrast reactions.

86. **Answer-a.** The treatment of cutaneous effects is largely dependent on the extent of the hives. If the patient develops only a few scattered hives, drug treatment probably is not necessary. The patient should be watched for other symptoms. If the patient is bothered by mild hives, an H_1-blocker antihistamine such as diphenhydramine (Benadryl) can be administered. Typical dosage is 25 to 50 mg given intravenously. Hives may become more prominent but may not be a component of a generalized systemic or anaphylactoid reaction. In these situations treatment consists of an H_2 blocker, such as cimetidine (Tagamet). Typical dosage is 300 mg intravenously, diluted and given slowly.

87. **Answer-a.** Oral or intravenous contrast agents fill certain structures with a higher density material, subsequently raising the structure's ability to attenuate the x-ray beam. It is important to note that the contrast agent does not change the body tissues but only resides in them.

88. **Answer-a.** Diabetes mellitus and associated renal insufficiency increase the patient's risk of progressive deterioration of renal func-

tion. Caution should be used before administering an iodinated contrast material in these patients.

89. **Answer-a.** Viscosity can be described as the thickness or friction of the fluid as it flows. The viscosity of contrast material can be significantly decreased by heating the liquid to body temperature. This heating facilitates rapid injection through small-bore needles and intravenous catheters.

90. **Answer-b.** The clearance of iodinated contrast media is primarily through the kidney by glomerular filtration. Under normal conditions nearly 100% of contrast material is excreted in this way. In patients with complete kidney failure, vicarious excretion (i.e., through the liver and gut) occurs.

91. **Answer-d.** All are factors that increase a patient's risk of experiencing an adverse reaction. Other factors also included in the guidelines are significant allergic history (not to drugs), poor hydration, diabetes mellitus, myelomatosis, youth, severe generalized debilitation, and acute anxiety.

92. **Answer-c.** The CT dose index (CTDI) is a measurement of radiation dose delivered by a specific CT system. It is reported by the scanners' manufacturers to the United States Food and Drug Administration and to prospective customers. Slice spacing must equal slice thickness for the resulting dose to be reported as the CTDI. If there is slice overlap or gap, the value is calculated to account for the difference, and the result is the multiple scan average dose (MSAD).

93. **Answer-b.** Iodinated contrast media can have a significant dehydrating effect on patients because of the difference in osmolality between the contrast media and body fluid. It follows that the newer contrast media, having an osmolality that is closer to that of body fluid, produce less patient dehydration.

94. **Answer-c.** Oral contrast material is important to differentiate fluid-filled bowel loops from a mass or abnormal fluid collection. There is no universally accepted oral contrast dose, and opinions vary widely within the field. It is accepted that, in general, more oral contrast is better, although patient compliance is often a limiting factor. Standard radiography suspensions cannot be used in CT because their high density produces an unacceptable amount of streak artifacts. These conventional agents cannot simply be diluted for use in CT because of their tendency to settle after ingestion.

95. **Answer-a.** A platelet count is often performed before a percutaneous biopsy procedure as a method of assessing the patient's risk of bleeding complications. The normal range for a platelet count is 250,000 to 450,000 cubic millimeters (mm^3).

96. **Answer-c.** Flow-control injectors are recommended for body scanning because a specified volume can be delivered at a specified rate. These factors can be recorded and reproduced in subsequent follow-up studies. Unfortunately, contrast extravasations and air embolus may still occur when using a flow-controlled injector, and, as with all forms of intravenous injection, safety precautions must be diligently followed.

97. **Answer-b.** Because the injection rate is often increased, the hand bolus method is an improvement over the drip method. However, consistency and reproducibility are not attainable, and a serious risk of operator radiation exposure exists.

98. **Answer-c.** The term *osmolality* refers to the number of particles in solution as compared with water. The classification ionic or nonionic refers to whether the molecules of the solution form ions in a water solution. Although many nonionic contrast agents have low osmolality, not all do. Hexabrix® is an example of a contrast medium that has low osmolality but is ionic.

99. **Answer-b.** Osmolality refers to the number of particles in solution as compared with water. Older, low-osmolality agents have up to seven times the number of particles in solution as water. The newer, low-osmolar agents have significantly less, but still contain approximately twice the particles in solution as body fluids. Studies show that newer contrast agents produce approximately one fifth as many reactions as the conventional contrast agents produced. Unfortunately, these newer contrast agents do not eliminate serious reactions, and fatal reactions may still occur. Studies have shown that nonionic contrast medium is less injurious to cutaneous and subcutaneous tissue than conventional high-osmolar contrast material.

100. **Answer-c.** Barium sulfate is an inert substance that passes through the body basically unchanged. Procedural complications to orally administered barium sulfate solution are rare and include aspiration pneumonitis, barium impaction, and intravasation.

101. **Answer-c.** Oral contrast agents can be delivered by means of a nasogastric tube. If vomiting is a problem, the contrast media can be dripped slowly into the nasogastric tube.

102. **Answer-c.** Intravenous catheters are recommended when repeated or continuous intravenous injections are administered. They consist of a needle that fits inside a flexible plastic catheter. This combination unit is inserted into the vein, and the catheter is advanced by slipping it forward over the needle.

103. **Answer-c**

104. **Answer-d.** If a major radiation exposure takes place during the first 10 days' post-conception, the most likely result is early intrauterine death. In the first trimester, the fetus is most vulnerable to radiation-induced congenital abnormalities. In the second and third trimester, a radiation exposure of 1 rad may significantly increase the risk of childhood leukemia.

105. **Answer-a.** The scan field of view determines the size of the fan beam, which, in turn, determines the number of detector cells that collect data. Figure 1–11 illustrates this concept.

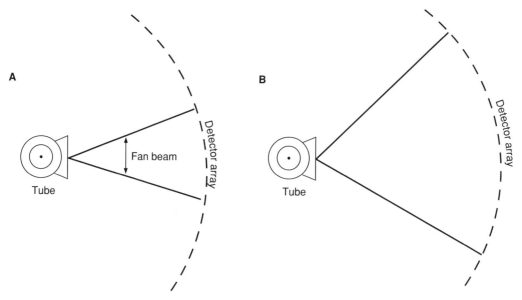

Figure 1-11. Increasing the scan field size will increase the number of detectors used to create the image. A *depicts a 25-cm scan field of view.* B *depicts a 42-cm scan field of view.*

106. **Answer-d.** Volume averaging, or partial volume effect, occurs when the beam attenuation values from more than one tissue type are averaged to produce a single pixel value. The amount of volume averaging present, therefore, depends on the size of the voxel. Of the listed factors, the only two that influence the voxel size are the matrix and the slice thickness. When a 10-mm slice is used, the z axis dimension, or depth of the voxel, is approximately 10 times longer than either the x or y direction. Therefore, the slice thickness contributes more significantly to volume averaging.

107. **Answer-c.** To create a CT image, the data must be broken down into small segments called pixels. Rows and columns of pixels comprise the matrix.

108. **Answer-a.** The denser the object the greater its beam attenuation ability. Because metals are denser than either fat or air, they have a higher capacity for beam attenuation.

109. **Answer-d.** The CT pioneer, Godfrey Newbold Hounsfield, developed a system to quantify beam attenuation. In this system, the attenuation capacity of water is 0, air is −1000, and bone is 1000. Objects with a beam attenuation less than that of water have an associated negative number. Conversely, substances with attenuations greater than that of water have a proportionally positive HU.

110. **Answer-c.** The components that produce x-rays are the x-ray tube and the anode. Both are housed in the gantry.

111. **Answer-a.** The ability of the tube to withstand the heat resulting from the production of x-rays is called heat capacity and is measured in million heat units (MHU).

112. **Answer-d.** Although exact rates vary on different scanners, the detectors on all systems are sampled very rapidly.

113. **Answer-d.** In a solid-state detector system, light is converted to an electric signal by the photodiode. In a xenon gas detector system, ionization of the gas produces an electric signal. In either case the electric current must be transformed into a format that is usable to the computer. Analog-to-digital converters in the CT system perform this function.

114. **Answer-a.** The phase of data acquisition comprises all the components necessary for creating x-rays and collecting data.

115. **Answer-c.** A third-generation scanner is the design that uses a detector array and a tube that produces a fan-shaped beam that covers the entire field of view. In the third-generation design, both the tube and detector array move in a circular path within the gantry. A fourth-generation scanner uses a detector array that is fixed in a 360° circle within the gantry. The tube rotates within the fixed detector array.

116. **Answer-c.** In the fourth-generation system, the x-ray source is closer to the detectors. All other things being equal, a somewhat lower technique can be used. This is in accordance with the inverse square law.

117. **Answer-a.** Filtering the x-ray beam removes long wavelength, or "soft," x-rays that do not contribute to the CT image but increase the patient's radiation dose. The second purpose of filtration is to reduce beam-hardening artifacts by creating a more uniform beam intensity.

118. **Answer-d.** One main type of detector is the xenon gas variety, which is kept under pressure in casings. The second type is made from solid-state crystals and gives off a brief flash of light when struck by x-rays; therefore, they are often referred to as scintillators.

119. **Answer-d.** Generally, more than 99% of the energy used in the creation of x-rays is lost as heat.

120. **Answer-c.** The raw data include all measurements obtained from the detector array. Typically only a portion of these data is used to create the actual image. The data that are selected for use in the image are referred to as image data.

121. **Answer-d.** Although a small tube filament provides better spatial resolution due to reduced penumbra, a trade-off is necessary because the smaller filament cannot tolerate high milliampere (mA) levels. Many systems contain two filament sizes, one for lower mA settings and a larger filament for settings over 200 mA.

122. **Answer-a.** A scan produced from a tube arc of 360° plus the width of the field of view is referred to as an overscan. Overscans are more common in fourth-generation scanner designs because the views acquired with these systems are not recorded instantaneously. This timing increases the inconsistency of data within views, and motion is more problematic. By allowing some overlap of data from the first and last tube positions, overscan reduces motion artifacts.

123. **Answer-c.** In a third-generation system the tube always rotates in conjunction with the detector arc. Whether the tube first rotates in one direction, then stops to rotate in the opposite direction as opposed to rotating in the same direction is not dependent on generation, but rather on whether the system contains a slip-ring device.

124. **Answer-a.** Any object smaller than a pixel is averaged in with the remainder of the pixel, thereby making it possible that the object goes undetected. Even assuming that the object is approximately the size of a pixel, random chance plays a role in whether the ob-

ject is detected on the image. To illustrate, assume that the object in question is a B-B, and it is approximately the same size as the pixel shown in Figure 1–12. Chance dictates whether the B-B falls entirely within the pixel as in diagram a, between two pixels as in diagram b, or at the intersection of four pixels as in diagram c. In these three cases, the image resulting from diagram a has the best chance of accurately displaying the B-B, whereas the image resulting from diagram c is least likely to display the object. The Nyquist sampling theorem accounts for this chance element by stating that the object has a better chance of detection if it is twice the size of the pixel or larger.

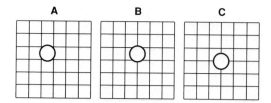

Figure 1-12. The Nyquist Sampling Theorem states that an object will have an increased opportunity of being resolved in the image if it is at least twice the size of a pixel.

125. **Answer-b.** Basically, the contrast–detail response states that if the technique is kept the same then as the object size decreases, its visibility diminishes. In addition, a small object is more readily visualized if it has a significantly different density than its background. An example of a high-density object is a calcified nodule in the lung. Although the nodule may be quite small, it has a greater chance of being visible on the image because its density varies sharply from the surrounding lung tissue. To summarize, assuming the technique remains unchanged, if the object's density remains the same and its size decreases, it is less visible on the image. If the object's size remains the same and its contrast increases, it is more visible on the image.

126. **Answer-a.** A grainy appearance on an image is most often referred to as noise, or quantum mottle. It is caused by insufficient x-ray photons reaching the detectors. Too low an mAs setting or overall low tube output results in too few x-rays being produced; subsequently, too few photons reach the detector.

127. **Answer-d.** Because all sources of x-rays contain photons of different energies, beam-hardening artifacts may occur. They result from lower-energy photons being preferentially absorbed, leaving only the higher-intensity photons to strike the detector array.

128. **Answer-b.** The range of pixel values can be determined by dividing in half the window width ($1600 \div 2 = 800$), subtracting the quotient from the window level to determine the lower limit ($-200 - 800 = -1000$), and then, to determine the upper limit, adding the quotient to the window level ($-200 + 800 = 600$).

129. **Answer-c.** The attenuation coefficient is a number derived from a specific strength beam that travels through a specific substance. Therefore, the density of the material being penetrated and the average photon energy of the beam are the only influencing factors.

130. **Answer-d.** On the Hounsfield scale, water is assigned the number 0. Because fat is less dense than water, it has a negative number.

131. **Answer-c.** The factors that directly affect the anode heat loading on a CT system are kilovolt-peak (kVp), mA setting, scan time, the number of sections, and the interscan delay time.

132. **Answer-c.** A decrease in matrix size increases the pixel size and, therefore, spatial resolution.

133. **Answer-b.** Adding filtration removes the low-energy, or "soft," photons from the beam. Removing the low-energy photons reduces scatter, thereby reducing patient radiation dose and improving image quality.

134. **Answer-b.** The number of detected photons is directly proportional to the slice thickness. Because a narrower slice thickness results in fewer photons striking the detector, the mAs must be increased to increase the number of photons, thereby maintaining image quality.

135. **Answer-c.** Within the x-ray tube, a filament is heated to "boil off" electrons. These electrons are then propelled across to strike the target material, resulting in the production of heat and x-rays.

136. **Answer-a.** The formula for determining pixel size is

$$\frac{\text{Field of view}}{\text{Matrix size}} = \text{Pixel size}$$

Make sure units for matrix and field size are the same. Therefore,

$$\frac{25 \text{ cm}}{512 \text{ mm}} = \frac{250 \text{ mm}}{512 \text{ mm}} = 0.488 \text{ mm, or rounded off } 0.5 \text{ mm}$$

137. **Answer-d.** If the structure is made of a variety of tissues with varying densities and this diversity lies within a single pixel, the system gives an averaged, rather than accurate CT number. This is the partial volume effect, or volume averaging. Choices 2, 3, and 4 each have an effect on the structure's ability to attenuate the x-ray beam and, therefore, have a direct effect on the assigned HU.

138. **Answer-d.** A narrow window limits the range of CT numbers displayed to provide greater discrimination between similar densities. A wide window encompasses a wide range of different tissue (e.g., displaying bone and lung) but does so at the expense of subtle density discrimination. Because the window setting is a display function that is set after the image has been acquired, it is impossible for it to affect any scanning parameter such as slice thickness and mAs. The appearance of quantum mottle can be decreased by widening the window width.

139. **Answer-a.** Beam-hardening artifacts are due to the x-ray beam possessing many different photon intensities. Filtration reduces the range of intensities by removing the low-intensity, or "soft," photons. Subsequently, adding x-ray beam filtration reduces beam-hardening artifacts.

140. **Answer-d.** The largest factor affecting visibility of low-contrast objects is the presence of noise in the image. Image noise results from too few photons reaching the detectors. The mA, scan time, and patient size all affect the number of photons that reach the detectors. The window setting affects the contrast scale, and the correct selection enhances the visibility of objects that vary only slightly from their background.

141. **Answer-c.** The generator produces high voltage and transmits it to the x-ray tube. A CT generator can have a single kVp or a variable kVp output. Tube output accuracy is more easily achieved in single kVp systems. A more sophisticated generator is required to produce accurate output with a variable kVp.

142. **Answer-a.** The display processor converts the digital reconstructed image into a gray scale image by assigning groups of HU to each shade of gray. This process allows the image to be displayed on the cathode-ray tube (CRT) monitor.

143. **Answer-a.** This process may also be described as retrospectively changing the data incrementation. Because a spiral scan acquires a volume of data, that data can be re-

constructed anywhere within the volume. For example, a 10-second spiral scan series is acquired with a slice thickness of 10 mm, and the first image contains data from table position 10–20; the data could be retrospectively reconstructed so that an image is produced from table position 15–25. Note that the slice thickness does not change, it remains 10 mm. Slice thickness is controlled by the collimator and cannot be altered retrospectively. Software in a spiral scan system can eliminate artifacts from table motion because the motion is predictable. It does not control patient movement artifacts.

144. **Answer-b.** Because raw data require much more computer space than image data, archiving devices are designed to store only image data.

145. **Answer-a.** Because the materials within the phantom are known, linearity can be checked by matching the CT numbers obtained from scanning to those known values. In a CT system with acceptable linearity, CT numbers plotted against the linear attenuation coefficient result in a straight line as shown in Figure 1-13.

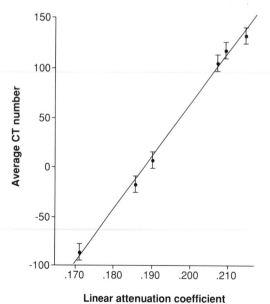

Figure 1-13. In a CT system with acceptable linearity, a straight line will result when numbers are plotted.

146. **Answer-d.** A sagittal reformation is obtained by stacking all available images and then creating a new image from a slice of data in the sagittal plane. To stack the images, they must possess the same parameters.

147. **Answer-a.** A unique advantage to three-dimensional image reconstruction is the ability to isolate a specific bone so that it can be viewed without the risk of nearby structures obscuring crucial information.

148. **Answer-c.** To retrospectively reconstruct an image in a different display field size, the raw data must still be available. To create a new image that includes more anatomy than the original, the scan field must be larger than the original display field size.

149. **Answer-a.** The shortened exam time permits a more effective, focused use of contrast media. Because scanning takes place with higher intravascular levels of contrast media, visualization of vessels is improved, and there is more intense parenchyma enhancement. This results in improved detection of pathology.

150. **Answer-c.** In contrast, the process by which the image is automatically processed during a routine scan procedure is often called prospective reconstruction.

Exam 2

Questions

1. In Figure 2–1 identify the structure indicated by arrow #1.

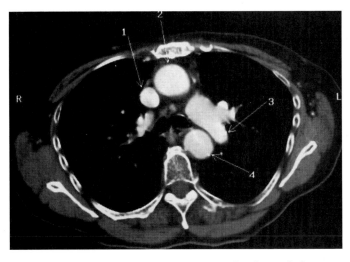

   a. ascending aorta   c. brachiocephalic artery
   b. superior vena cava   d. right atrium

2. In Figure 2–1 identify the structure indicated by arrow #2.

   a. ascending aorta
   b. superior vena cava
   c. right pulmonary artery
   d. right ventricle

3. In Figure 2–1 identify the structure indicated by arrow #3.

   a. descending aorta
   b. subclavian artery
   c. left atrium
   d. left pulmonary artery

4. In Figure 2–1 identify the structure indicated by arrow #4.

   a. descending aorta
   b. inferior vena cava
   c. portal vein
   d. left atrium

5. What can be done to distend the pyriform sinuses on a computed tomography (CT) image?

   a. Have the patient perform a modified Valsalva maneuver.
   b. Have the patient hyperextend the neck.
   c. Have the patient use a steroid nasal spray before scanning.
   d. Use a spiral scan technique.

6. An overscan can be defined as a scan

    a. produced from 360° of tube travel plus approximately the width of the field of view
    b. produced from 180° of tube travel plus the degree of arc from the fan angle
    c. that utilizes a higher radiation dose than is necessary to produce an adequate image
    d. in which a portion of the patient's anatomy does not lie entirely within the scan field of view

7. The inferior extent of a routine brain scan is the

    a. vertex
    b. foramen magnum
    c. clivus
    d. sella turcica

8. The slice thickness in Figure 2–2 is 1 mm. Figure 2–2 is from what type of study?

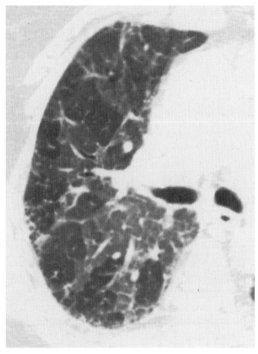

    a. spiral chest
    b. routine chest
    c. high-resolution chest CT
    d. dissecting thoracic aneurysm examination

9. All of the following could be a clinical indication for obtaining the image in Figure 2–2 EXCEPT

    a. metastatic disease
    b. asbestosis
    c. emphysema
    d. interstitial disease

10. Which technique can be used to reduce streak artifacts on images of the lower neck?

    a. Decrease milliampere-seconds (mAs).
    b. Lift the patient's arms over his head.
    c. Instruct the patient to lower his shoulders as much as possible.
    d. Place the patient in a prone position.

11. When scanning the thorax, the use of a spiral or cluster scan technique reduces

    a. slice misregistration
    b. radiation dose to the patient
    c. the tube heat loading
    d. image noise

12. In Figure 2–3, arrow #1 depicts

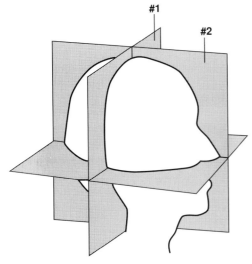

#1
#2

    a. a coronal plane
    b. a central plane
    c. a sagittal plane
    d. an axial plane

13. In Figure 2–3, arrow #2 depicts

    a. an axial plane
    b. a ventral plane
    c. a sagittal plane
    d. a coronal plane

14. What is the result when image data are manipulated retrospectively to produce images in a different plane?

    a. retrospective reconstructions
    b. reformatted images
    c. z-axis data shifted images
    d. perpendicular display field

15. Contrast flow rate is not critical for detecting pathology in which organ?

    a. brain
    b. liver
    c. neck
    d. chest

16. In which situation would intravenous contrast be particularly valuable for scanning the thorax?

    a. to rule out interstitial disease
    b. if the patient possesses insufficient mediastinal fat
    c. to localize a calcified nodule in the lung
    d. to evaluate pneumonia

17. Which part of the sphenoid bone supports the pons and carries the abducent nerve?

    a. greater wing
    b. lesser wing
    c. dorsum sellae
    d. superior turbinate

18. The most common extracranial solid malignant neoplasms of childhood, accounting for approximately 10% of all pediatric neoplasms, are

    a. sarcomas
    b. Osgood-Schlatter tumors
    c. neuroblastomas
    d. hemangiomas

19. In Figure 2–4 identify the structure indicated by arrow #1.

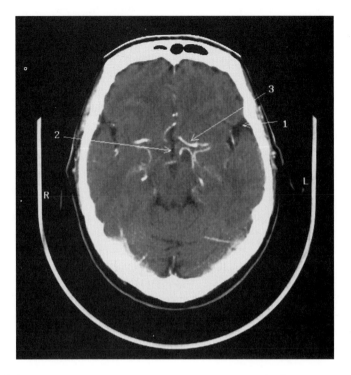

a. falx cerebri

b. cerebral aqueduct

c. central sulcus

d. sylvian fissure

20. In Figure 2–4 identify the structure indicated by arrow #2.

a. midbrain

b. choroidal fissure

c. third ventricle

d. fourth ventricle

21. In Figure 2–4 identify the structure indicated by arrow #3.

a. anterior cerebral artery

b. middle cerebral artery

c. tentorium cerebelli

d. thalamostriate vein

22. What divides the abdomen into dorsal and ventral compartments?

a. diaphragmatic crus

b. falciform ligament

c. retroperitoneal fascia

d. Gerota fascia

23. Which of the following is the key concept when performing a CT study of the pancreas?

    a. Scanning should be performed in the equilibrium phase of intravenous contrast enhancement.
    b. Oral contrast must be administered at least 4 hours before scanning.
    c. Identification of all structures adjacent to the pancreas should be performed by the use of oral and intravenous media.
    d. Contrast medium may mask adjacent structures; therefore, scanning should be performed without intravenous or oral agents.

24. Spaces on the interior of the cranium that produce grooves on the inner surface of the bones and are venous channels along which the blood runs in its passage back from the brain are called

    a. cavities
    b. ventricles
    c. foramina
    d. sinuses

25. Which of the following is necessary for a CT system to produce spiral scans?

    a. third-generation design
    b. fourth-generation design
    c. gantry with a slip-ring design
    d. 1-second tube rotation

26. Which disadvantage occurs when body scans are performed in the bolus phase of contrast enhancement?

    a. Lesions may reach equilibrium with surrounding tissue and be undetectable.
    b. The volume of contrast necessary is twice that needed for other phases.
    c. The venous structures are not yet opacified and may be difficult to differentiate from low attention lesions.
    d. A mechanical injector cannot be used.

27. Osteomyelitis can be defined as

    a. inflammation of bone, particularly the marrow, that is caused by a pathogenic organism
    b. softening of the bone caused from a deficiency of vitamin D
    c. any disease process that results in the reduction in the mass of bone per unit of volume
    d. the presence of bone-containing nodules in the skin

28. Figure 2–5 is from a study in which the patient was given

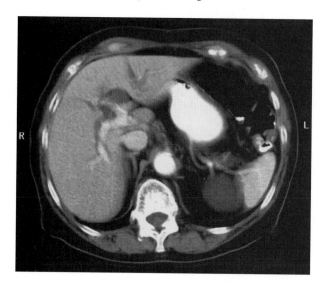

a. oral contrast only

b. intravenous contrast only

c. oral and intravenous contrast

d. oral, intravenous, and intrathecal contrast

29. One of the abnormalities displayed in Figure 2–5 is

a. aortic aneurysm

b. esophageal varices

c. fatty infiltrate of the liver

d. biliary obstruction

30. What divides the liver into two main lobes?

a. common hepatic artery

b. falciform ligament

c. celiac axis

d. hepatic muscle

31. The long, flat muscle that extends anteriorly along the entire length of the abdomen is the

a. obturator internus muscle

b. psoas muscle

c. quadratus lumborum muscle

d. rectus abdominus muscle

32. The brachiocephalic artery bifurcates into the

a. right common carotid and right subclavian arteries

b. internal and external carotid arteries

c. left common carotid and left vertebral arteries

d. superior and inferior mesenteric arteries

33. Which ducts join to form the common bile duct?

a. Bartholin duct and alveolar duct

b. efferent duct and Stensen duct

c. pancreatic duct and renal duct

d. cystic duct and hepatic duct

34. Trauma, tumor, and birth defects are the three most common indications for

a. high-resolution chest CT

b. CT angiography

c. CT portography

d. three-dimensional image reformation

35. A coronal sinus study is completed with the patient in the prone position. The technologist has neglected to input the correct position, and the computer defaults to the supine scanning position. What is the result of this error?

1. incorrect pixel values
2. incorrect left–right annotation of the image
3. incorrect anterior–posterior annotation of the image
4. excessive image noise

    a. 2 only
    b. 2 and 3
    c. 1, 2, and 3
    d. 1, 2, 3, and 4

36. To produce multiplanar reformations, which of the following factors must be consistent on all cross-sectional slices?

1. image center
2. gantry tilt
3. slice thickness
4. mAs

    a. 1 and 2
    b. 2 and 3
    c. 1, 3, and 4
    d. 2, 3, and 4

37. In Figure 2–6 identify the structure indicated by arrow #1.

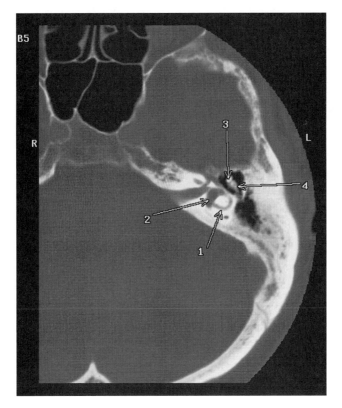

    a. petrosal nerve canal
    b. vestibular aqueduct

    c. lateral semicircular canal
    d. epitympanic recess

38. In Figure 2–6 identify the structure indicated by arrow #2.

    a. internal jugular vein
    b. round window
    c. mastoid antrum
    d. vestibule

39. In Figure 2–6 identify the structure indicated by arrow #3.

    a. cochlea
    b. vidian canal
    c. malleus
    d. stapes

40. In Figure 2–6 identify the structure indicated by arrow #4.

    a. incus
    b. malleus
    c. facial nerve
    d. eustachian tube

41. A neoplasm that is composed of immature, undifferentiated cells is often called a

    a. lipoma
    b. melanoma
    c. blastoma
    d. carcinogen

42. The process by which scans are acquired quickly, at the same table position, after a rapid bolus injection of intravenous contrast material is called

    a. spiral scanning
    b. high-resolution CT
    c. nonincremental dynamic scanning
    d. CT angiography

43. Respiratory misregistration can be reduced by which of the following techniques?

    1. using a soft, or low-contrast, algorithm
    2. administering oxygen to the patient before scanning
    3. using a spiral scan technique
    4. clustering axial scans in groups of three or more
    a. 1 only
    b. 2 only
    c. 1 and 4
    d. 3 and 4

44. The display function that creates a bar graph to show how frequently a range of CT numbers occurs within a specified region of interest is called

    a. a gray scale
    b. an image correlation graph
    c. a histogram
    d. a beam attenuation chart

45. A doublefold of peritoneum that is attached to the stomach and connects it with the abdominal viscera is called the

    a. aryepiglottic fold
    b. omentum
    c. lumbar plexus
    d. lateroconal fascia

46. The area starting at the midportion of the eighth thoracic vertebra to the bottom of the eleventh thoracic vertebra is a rough guideline for estimating the location of the

    a. carina
    b. aortic bifurcation
    c. pancreas
    d. left ventricle

47. The patient is lying prone with his neck hyperextended, and the gantry is angled cephalad. The study being performed is a

    a. paranasal sinuses
    b. larynx
    c. cervical spine
    d. posterior fossa

48. What passes through the optic canal?

    1. optic nerve
    2. ophthalmic artery
    3. anterior cerebral artery
    4. medial rectus muscle

       a. 1 only
       b. 1 and 2
       c. 1 and 3
       d. 2 and 4

49. How can the operator broaden the range of visible CT numbers on an image?

    a. Increase the mAs setting.
    b. Switch to a smaller focal spot.
    c. Increase the window width setting.
    d. Warm the x-ray tube before scanning.

50. In Figure 2–7 identify the structure indicated by arrow #1.

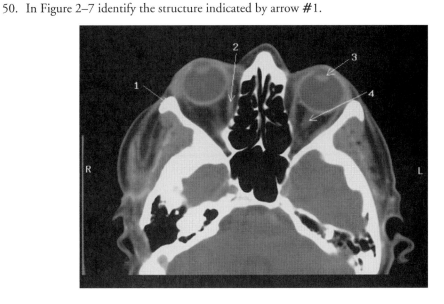

    a. anterior clinoid
    b. greater wing of sphenoid

    c. zygoma
    d. medial wall of maxilla

51. In Figure 2–7 identify the structure indicated by arrow **#2.**

    a. superior oblique muscle
    b. superior ophthalmic vein
    c. optic nerve
    d. medial rectus muscle

52. In Figure 2–7 identify the structure indicated by arrow **#3.**

    a. lens
    b. cornea
    c. vitreous humor
    d. sclera

53. In Figure 2–7 identify the structure indicated by arrow **#4.**

    a. medial rectus muscle
    b. optic nerve
    c. ophthalmic vein
    d. anterior cerebral artery

54. Which of the following is a generally accepted principle concerning the administration of intravenous iodinated contrast materials for body scanning?

    a. Spiral scanning requires approximately 33% more intravenous contrast media than conventional scanning methods.
    b. Scans of the liver should be performed in the equilibrium phase.
    c. Bolus injections are preferable to drip infusions.
    d. Contrast medium flow rate is much more important than the time of the delay between injection and scanning.

55. In Figure 2–8 identify the structure indicated by arrow #1.

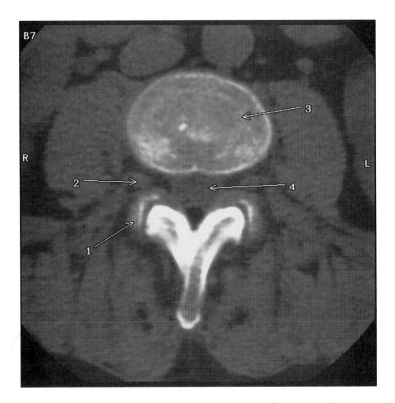

a. ligamentum flavum
b. superior articular process (L4)

c. inferior articular process (L3)
d. lamina

56. In Figure 2–8 identify the structure indicated by arrow #2.

a. nerve ganglion
b. dural sac
c. vertebral artery
d. basivertebral veins

57. In Figure 2–8 identify the structure indicated by arrow #3.

a. intervertebral disk (L3–L4)
b. intervertebral foramen
c. pedicle
d. quadratus lumborum muscle

58. In Figure 2–8 identify the structure indicated by arrow #4.

a. nerve root
b. ligamentum flavum
c. dural sac
d. annulus

59. A melanoma is found in

a. the bone marrow
b. a skin mole
c. the inner ear
d. the meninges of the brain

60. How is an optical disk labeled if it cannot be reused?

   a. analog only
   b. digital only
   c. MOD
   d. WORM

61. In Figure 2–9 identify the structure indicated by arrow #1.

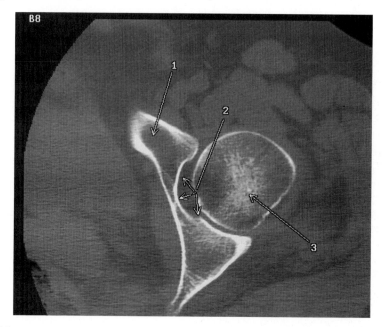

   a. ischium
   b. greater trochanter

   c. anterior–inferior iliac spine
   d. pubis

62. In Figure 2–9 identify the structure indicated by arrow #2.

   a. acetabulum
   b. obturator foramen
   c. symphysis pubis
   d. superior pubic ramus

63. In Figure 2–9 identify the structure indicated by arrow #3.

   a. pubis
   b. ischium
   c. head of femur
   d. psoas muscle

64. In scanning the brain, using which one of the following reference lines reduces the radiation exposure to the lens of the eye?

   a. acanthomeatal line
   b. orbital meatal line
   c. glabellomeatal line
   d. infraorbital meatal line

65. The term goiter refers to

    a. a malignant, highly metastatic tumor of the thyroid gland
    b. an endocrine disorder caused by failure of the ovaries to respond to the pituitary hormone, gonadotropin
    c. a hormone secreted by the anterior lobe of the pituitary that stimulates the thyroid gland
    d. an enlargement of the thyroid gland

66. In Figure 2–10 identify the structure indicated by arrow #1.

    a. acromion
    b. head of the humerus
    c. head of the femur
    d. brachial plexus

67. In Figure 2–10 identify the structure indicated by arrow #2.

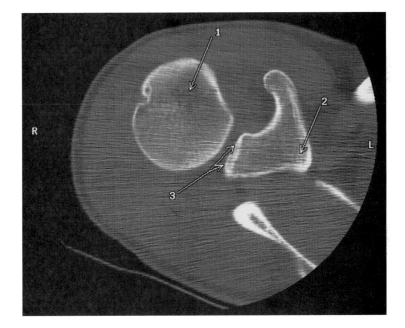

    a. scapula
    b. second rib
    c. clavicle
    d. lesser tubercle

68. In Figure 2–10 identify the structure indicated by arrow #3.

    a. deltoid fossa
    b. coronoid notch
    c. glenoid fossa
    d. acromion

69. The absence or impairment of the ability to communicate through speech, writing, or signs due to dysfunction of the brain centers is called

    a. aphagia
    b. aphonia
    c. apheresis
    d. aphasia

70. In a spiral scan procedure the pitch is set at 2 (2:1) and the slice thickness is set at 10 mm. How far does the table travel in 1 second?

   a. 5 mm
   b. 10 mm
   c. 15 mm
   d. 20 mm

71. In Figure 2–11 identify the structure indicated by arrow #1.

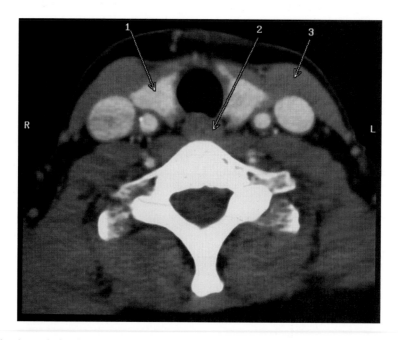

   a. right thyroid gland
   b. thyroid cartilage

   c. vocal cords
   d. strap muscle

72. In Figure 2–11 identify the structure indicated by arrow #2.

   a. paratracheal mass
   b. esophagus
   c. nuchal ligament
   d. glottic space

73. In Figure 2–11 identify the structure indicated by arrow #3.

   a. trapezius muscle
   b. sternocleidomastoid muscle
   c. rhomboid muscle
   d. left lobe of the thyroid

74. Which of the following are true statements concerning iodinated water-soluble agents?

    1. Their use is based on their therapeutic and pharmacological actions.
    2. They are nearly isotonic.
    3. Their use is based on their distribution in and elimination from the body.
    4. Histamines are responsible for the majority of the hemodynamic, cardiac, and subjective effects.
       a. 2 only
       b. 3 only
       c. 2, 3, and 4
       d. 1, 2, 3, and 4

75. What is the normal range of creatinine values?

    a. 0.7–1.4 mg/dl
    b. 2.5–3.5 mg/dl
    c. 10–20 mg/dl
    d. 20–30 mg/dl

76. What category of drug stimulates the sympathetic nervous system causing constriction of blood vessels, increased cardiac output, an increase in blood pressure, and relaxation of smooth muscle lining of the respiratory tract?

    a. vasodilators, such as Sorbitrate and Apresoline
    b. anticholinergics, such as atropine and scopolamine
    c. adrenergics, such as epinephrine and isoproterenol
    d. diuretics, such as Lasix and Diuril

77. What is the peak time for urinary excretion of contrast media following intravenous injection?

    a. 1.0 minute
    b. 1.5 minutes
    c. 3.0 minutes
    d. 5.0 minutes

78. In which one of the following classifications do contrast reactions require an immediate response? Symptoms may be pulmonary and laryngeal edema along with a prolonged decrease in blood pressure, cardiac arrhythmias, and cardiac arrest.

    a. minor reactions
    b. moderate reactions
    c. major reactions
    d. idiopathic reactions

79. The laboratory value prothrombin time (PT) is used for

    a. determining the dosages of anticoagulant drugs
    b. identifying deficiencies in coagulation factors, prothrombin and fibrinogen
    c. determining the number of circulating platelets in venous or arterial blood
    d. measuring the time of platelet clot formation after a small puncture wound

80. The term diaphoretic describes a patient who

    a. is feverish with hot, dry skin
    b. is sweating profusely with pale, cool skin
    c. is having difficulty breathing
    d. has red, raised welts on her skin from an allergic response

81. The advancing pressure wave in an artery that is caused by the expulsion of blood when the left ventricle of the heart contracts is called

    a. a blood pressure
    b. a P wave
    c. a pulse
    d. an arrhythmia

82. A patient that is suffering from dyspnea has

    a. difficulty urinating
    b. difficulty breathing
    c. an insulin deficiency
    d. blood-tinged sputum

83. The respiratory rate of children is

    a. more sporadic than adults
    b. nearly identical to adults
    c. faster than adults
    d. slower than adults

84. If a patient's pulse is described as "thready," it means

    a. the volume of blood is high, but the force it exerts is low
    b. the patient is experiencing tachycardia
    c. the heart has been artificially stimulated, probably by drugs or exertion
    d. it is weak and irregular

85. It is important to take a blood pressure reading

    a. on any outpatient that is to receive intravenous contrast medium or systemic medication
    b. on all CT patients
    c. on any patient with a history of hypertension
    d. after the intravenous injection of a contrast medium

86. What is the proper method of disposing of a used syringe?

    a. Recap needle, then remove from syringe to dispose of in a Sharps container.
    b. Break the needle off the syringe, then dispose of in a Sharps container.
    c. Provided the needle is recapped, dispose of in a regular trash container.
    d. Dispose of the syringe and needle in a Sharps container without recapping.

87. According to the Centers for Disease Control, the single, most effective way to prevent the spread of disease is by

    a. surgical aseptic techniques
    b. autoclaving all equipment used for health care
    c. frequent hand washing
    d. using a bleach solution to clean patient care equipment

88. What is the most common side effect of diphenhydramine hydrochloride?

    a. tachycardia
    b. drowsiness
    c. nausea or vomiting
    d. hives

89. Which of the following is a true statement concerning contrast reactions?

    a. Contrast media reactions always cause elevated plasma histamine values.
    b. Significant increases in plasma histamine values never occur in patients experiencing a contrast media reaction.
    c. Premedication with drugs such as prednisone or diphenhydramine eliminates a contrast reaction in all patients.
    d. The exact mechanism of anaphylactoid reactions to iodinated contrast media is unknown.

90. If an intravascular drug is described as *isotonic*, it

   a. has been dissolved in a normal saline solution
   b. is at body temperature
   c. has nearly the same number of particles in solution as body fluids
   d. has molecules that form ions in a water solution

91. Which of the following is a primary characteristic responsible for a contrast material's hemodynamic, cardiac, and subjective effects?

   a. ionic nature
   b. biexponential decay curve
   c. acute lethal dose (LD_{50})
   d. osmolality

92. The patient's radiation dose for an average CT study is expressed by which calculation?

   a. quality factor
   b. sievert (Sv) per mm of exposed tissue
   c. multiple scan average dose (MSAD)
   d. dose of single slice times number of slices

93. Concerning the patient radiation dose, which of the following is a *true* statement?

   a. Because the x-ray source rotates around the patient, the center of the patient receives only one-hundredth of the radiation exposure as that of the skin.
   b. In a CT study, there is no scatter outside the designated slice.
   c. The difference between entrance exposure and exit exposure is much greater in CT than in conventional film/screen radiography.
   d. Radiation doses for CT examinations are substantially higher than those for film/screen studies of the same body part.

94. Obtaining written consent from the patient before the injection of an iodinated contrast material serves what purpose?

   a. protects the hospital and health care worker from litigation if an adverse reaction should develop
   b. reduces the likelihood of an adverse reaction because patient anxiety concerning the examination is reduced
   c. provides documentation that the procedure and associated risks were discussed with the patient before the examination
   d. ensures that, should an adverse reaction occur, arbitration is used rather than litigation

95. Concerning skin preparation for a biopsy procedure, what is required before the removal of hair?

   a. Blood urea nitrogen (BUN) and creatinine values are known to be within the normal range.
   b. A physician has ordered hair removal.
   c. The skin has been cleansed and a sterile drape has been placed.
   d. The patient is premedicated with a sedative.

96. A patient who is scheduled for a CT examination of the abdomen and pelvis should follow which preparations?

   1. refrain from eating 2 hours before the examination
   2. refrain from liquids (except the oral contrast required) beginning at midnight before the examination
   3. drink oral contrast following the guidelines specified by the facility
   4. discontinue any medications beginning at midnight before the examination

   a. 1 and 2
   b. 1 and 3
   c. 3 and 4
   d. 1, 2, 3, and 4

97. What causes barium peritonitis?

    a. aspiration of barium into the lungs

    b. the administration of a large volume of oral barium sulfate in patients with an obstructed bowel

    c. barium leaking into the peritoneal cavity from a perforation of the gastrointestinal tract

    d. too large a dose of an oral barium sulfate suspension in a patient with renal insufficiency

98. Drip infusion method of delivering contrast media may

    a. mask abnormalities that would have been detected without contrast

    b. be easily regulated by injecting air into the bottle

    c. be regulated by setting the bottle height identically for each patient

    d. result in flow rates of over 3 ml/sec

99. What is the correct cycle of compressions and breaths when delivering cardiopulmonary resuscitation (CPR) to a child?[1]

    a. 5 compressions, then 1 breath

    b. 10 compressions, then 2 breaths

    c. 15 compressions, then 2 breaths

    d. 20 compressions, then 3 breaths

100. What injection site is typically best for pediatric patients that receive a bolus of contrast?

    a. antecubital site

    b. posterior hand

    c. digital vein

    d. interosseous vein

101. Regarding the fetal risk when exposing a pregnant woman to radiation, all of the following are true EXCEPT

    a. The risk of congenital malformation increases at doses greater than 10 rads.

    b. If exposed after 150 days' postconception, the greatest effect is an increased risk of childhood malignancies.

    c. Regardless of the dose, an abortion to avoid the possibility of radiation-induced congenital anomalies is considered whenever a pregnant women is exposed to radiation from a medical source.

    d. If exposure occurs at 50 to 70 days' postconception, the most likely abnormalities are growth and mental retardation.

102. A bluish color to the skin, mouth, gums, and nail beds is a sign of what condition?

    a. radiation poisoning

    b. critically low blood sugar

    c. cerebral vascular accident

    d. respiratory distress

103. What technique provides the best opportunity for scanning when the intravenous contrast medium is in the bolus phase?

    a. deliver 150 ml of contrast at a rate of 2 ml/sec; start spiral scanning at the same time the contrast medium is started

    b. deliver 100 ml of contrast at a rate of 2 ml/sec; start spiral scanning at 30 seconds after the initiation of contrast

    c. deliver 200 ml of contrast at a rate of 0.2 ml/sec; start spiral scanning 3 minutes after the initiation of contrast

    d. deliver 150 ml of contrast at a rate of 5 ml/sec; start spiral scanning 5 minutes after the initiation of contrast

[1]The American National Red Cross: *American Red Cross CPR Instructor's Manual.* 1988, p 260.

104. What is a contraindication to percutaneous biopsy?

    a. iodine allergy
    b. bleeding disorder
    c. sickle-cell anemia
    d. chronic obstructive pulmonary disease (COPD)

105. A disadvantage of spiral, or helical, scanning is

    a. it increases the partial volume effect
    b. multiplanar and three-dimensional reformations are not as good as those made with conventional scans
    c. it places a greater stress on the x-ray tube than conventional scans
    d. radiation exposure to the patient is nearly doubled

106. Beam-hardening artifacts are a result of

    a. the Nyquist effect
    b. the fact that x-rays are polychromatic in nature
    c. the fact that tissue densities are averaged to produce one less accurate pixel reading
    d. the fact that after being struck by an x-ray photon, detectors exhibit a brief afterglow

107. The y axis refers to

    a. the width of the pixel
    b. the height of the pixel
    c. the slice thickness
    d. the rotational nature of the x-ray tube

108. Beam attenuation can be defined as

    a. the phenomenon by which artifacts result from lower-energy photons being preferentially absorbed, leaving higher-intensity photons to strike the detector array
    b. x-ray energy that is produced from the sudden stoppage of electrons
    c. the ability of the detector to capture transmitted photons and change them to electronic signals
    d. the phenomenon by which an x-ray beam passing through a structure is decreased in intensity or amount because of absorption and interaction with matter

109. In a CT image the shade of gray that represents a particular structure is dependent on all of the following EXCEPT the

    a. gray scale
    b. density of the structure
    c. mAs
    d. intensity (hardness) of the x-ray as it emerges from the tube

110. Which of the following is a true statement concerning Hounsfield units (HU)?

    a. Inaccuracies in HU can be caused by volume averaging, artifacts, or improper equipment maintenance.
    b. HUs are absolute and can only be altered by changing the density of a measured structure.
    c. An HU is defined as the amount of energy required to raise the temperature of 1 g of water from 14.5°C to 15.5°C.
    d. Changing the window width or window setting alters the HU of a particular structure.

111. Which of the following is an equivalent of 1 milliampere (mA)?

    a. one millionth of an ampere
    b. one thousandth of an ampere
    c. a thousand amperes
    d. a million amperes

112. The ability of the tube to rid itself of heat is called

    a. heat capacity
    b. heat dissipation
    c. thermal potential
    d. thermal distribution

113. Which of the following converts the light emitted by the detector material into an electric current?

    a. data acquisition system (DAS)
    b. array processor
    c. photodiode
    d. analog-to-digital converter (ADC)

114. Which part of the CT system is responsible for converting the digitized data into shades of gray?

    a. photodiode
    b. array processor
    c. display processor
    d. analog-to-digital converter

115. Why is it necessary to convert the digitized data from the reconstruction processor to shades of gray?

    a. to allow HU to be assigned to each structure
    b. to remove streak artifacts from the final image
    c. to enhance the desirable aspects of the image and suppress the undesirable aspects
    d. so that an image can be displayed on the cathode-ray tube (CRT) monitor and recorded on film

116. Which of the following is an advantage of a CT system that can produce a variable kilo-volt-peak (kVp) output over the type that produces a single kVp output? Variable kVp systems

    a. are less expensive
    b. offer higher mA settings, which subsequently allow a reduction in scan times
    c. have less maintenance problems and, therefore, experience less down time
    d. allow for an increased capacity to discriminate between different tissues

117. Figure 2–12 illustrates a scanner with a

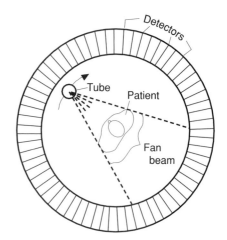

    a. second-generation design
    b. third-generation design
    c. fourth-generation design
    d. fifth-generation design

118. What is the purpose of a bow tie filter?

    a. increases the speed of the striking photons
    b. prevents aliasing artifacts
    c. improves detector efficiency
    d. reduces the beam intensity at the periphery of the beam, corresponding to the thinner area of a patient's anatomy

119. Slice thickness is *primarily* determined by

 a. focal spot size
 b. distance between detectors
 c. source collimator
 d. matrix size

120. Ceramic rare earth, cesium iodide, cadmium tungstate, and bismuth germinate are all examples of materials used to make

 a. intravenous or oral contrast agents
 b. solid-state detectors
 c. computer chips
 d. beam filtration

121. The process of converting the data from the attenuation profile to a matrix is known as

 a. convolution
 b. archiving
 c. back projection
 d. referencing

122. Which one of the following statements is true concerning raw data?

 a. Raw data are necessary to change the display field size (zoom, target) after the study has been completed.
 b. Raw data must be available to create multiplanar reformations.
 c. To obtain a Hounsfield measurement on a structure, raw data must be available.
 d. Three-dimensional models are created with raw data.

123. What effect does increasing the size of the pixel have on spatial resolution?

 a. decreases spatial resolution
 b. increases spatial resolution in a linear manner
 c. increases spatial resolution in a nonlinear manner
 d. has no effect on spatial resolution

124. In general, which of the following is more of a problem with third-generation CT systems than with fourth-generation systems?

 a. increased scatter acceptance in the detector array
 b. more ring artifacts
 c. motion artifacts
 d. sampling artifacts

125. Which of the following factors affect spatial resolution?

 1. field of view
 2. slice thickness
 3. focal spot size
 4. modulation transfer function (MTF)
 a. 1 and 3
 b. 2 and 4
 c. 1, 2, and 4
 d. 1, 2, 3, and 4

126. Low-contrast resolution can be defined as the ability to

 a. produce a satisfactory image with a low radiation dose
 b. represent small objects and differentiate between closely spaced objects
 c. reproduce with accuracy a high-contrast edge
 d. distinguish objects with similar densities

127. How does radiation dose affect image noise?

 a. Radiation dose is proportional to image noise.
 b. Radiation dose has an inverse effect on image noise.
 c. As radiation dose decreases, noise decreases, but the noise decrease is not linear, rather it is dependent on factors such as tube heat and patient size.
 d. Radiation dose has no effect on image noise.

128. A streak artifact caused by a significant difference in density between contrast and air is called

   a. an air–contrast interface artifact
   b. a sampling artifact
   c. a beam-hardening artifact
   d. a ring artifact

129. Scan thickness is *primarily* important for the part it plays in

   a. noise reduction
   b. the contrast scale
   c. detector aperture opening
   d. volume averaging

130. Which of the following are advantages of a wide window setting?

   1. suppresses the display of image noise
   2. provides greater density discrimination between similar density objects
   3. encompasses greater anatomic diversity
   4. highlights the difference between the gray and white matter of the brain
   a. 1 and 2
   b. 1 and 3
   c. 2 and 3
   d. 1, 3, and 4

131. On a CT image of the brain, an area is measured, and its CT number, or HU, is 70. It is most likely composed of

   a. calcium
   b. air
   c. water
   d. fresh blood

132. On a CT image a structure is measured, and its CT number, or HU, is 1000. It is most likely

   a. bone
   b. air in the sinus
   c. a cyst
   d. fat

133. In the detectors in a CT system, geometric efficiency is controlled primarily by

   a. detector material (solid-state crystals or xenon gas chambers)
   b. type of photodiode used
   c. filtration
   d. detector spacing and aperture

134. The part of the CT system referred to as DAS is responsible for

   a. converting the light emitted from the detector to an electric current
   b. projecting the data from the attenuation profile onto a matrix
   c. sampling each of the detector cells many times per second
   d. converting digitized data to shades of gray to be displayed

135. X-rays are produced

   a. by manipulating light photons by means of a rotating anode
   b. from a rapid acceleration of target electrons
   c. from the sudden stoppage of fast moving electrons
   d. as a by-product in the creation of isotopes

136. A device for data storage that can be erased and reused is often referred to as

    a. MOD
    b. random access memory (RAM)
    c. WORM
    d. UNIX

137. Which factors may reduce the accuracy of a CT number (HU)?

    1. partial volume effect
    2. mAs
    3. generator size
    4. beam hardening
        a. 1 and 2
        b. 1 and 4
        c. 2 and 3
        d. 1, 2, 3, and 4

138. Why is tungsten used for the target material of most x-ray tubes?

    a. It has a high atomic number.
    b. It dissipates heat gradually.
    c. It is very stable; therefore, electrons cannot be dislodged, even when struck directly.
    d. It produces 99% characteristic x-rays.

139. The central processing unit (CPU) performs what function?

    a. long-term raw data storage
    b. short-term image data storage
    c. basic arithmetic and logical operations
    d. samples the detectors

140. All other factors being constant, what is the effect of decreasing the CT image matrix from 512^2 to 256^2?

    a. Patient dose increases.
    b. Gray scale expands for image display.
    c. Spatial resolution worsens.
    d. X-ray tube loading increases.

141. How many CT numbers are assigned to each pixel in the image matrix?

    a. one half the number of all values recorded from the detector array
    b. one
    c. the square root of the median value of each pixel
    d. 2 values for a 256^2 matrix; 4 values for a 512^2 matrix

142. Keeping all other factors constant, increasing the pitch from 1 to 2 (1:1 to 2:1) results in

    a. less anatomy being covered
    b. increased spatial resolution
    c. increased radiation dose to the patient
    d. widening of the effective slice thickness

143. Why is interpolation required to reconstruct a spiral CT image?

    a. so the tube can rotate continually in the same direction
    b. to "unslant" the individual slice because the slice beginning does not exactly match the slice end
    c. to compress the enormous amount of raw data produced
    d. to improve the heat dissipation rate

144. Metallic materials such as dental fillings, surgical clips, and prosthetic devices produce

    a. ring artifacts
    b. cupping artifacts
    c. streak artifacts
    d. image noise

145. A water phantom is scanned, and the standard deviation for a region of interest is obtained from the resulting image. This can be used to evaluate

    a. linearity
    b. noise
    c. spatial resolution
    d. slice thickness accuracy

146. A phantom contains two small objects, and the precise distance between them is known. The phantom is scanned, and the distance between the objects is measured using the distance feature available on the scanner. This test indicates

    a. noise
    b. slice thickness accuracy
    c. spatial resolution
    d. image distortion

147. The type of reformation by which individual slices are combined and smoothed so that their merged surfaces resemble the intact patient structure is

    a. coronal reformation
    b. ray–sum projection
    c. three-dimensional reformation
    d. maximum intensity projection

148. An area is scanned, and the resulting image appears too small on the CRT monitor. What is necessary to enlarge the image on the monitor and improve the spatial resolution?

    a. The raw data must be available.
    b. The system must have a magnification option.
    c. The scan field must be larger than the current display field.
    d. The patient must be rescanned using a smaller scan field of view.

149. What is necessary to be able to change the algorithm on a sinus image from standard to bone?

    a. Window width must be over 200.
    b. Display field must equal scan field.
    c. Raw data must be available.
    d. Study must have been acquired in a conventional axial method (not spiral).

150. Why would a 1.5 pitch be used on a vascular study that is primarily to be used to create a three-dimensional model?

    a. to allow the use of a lower concentration of iodinated contrast media
    b. to create wider slices
    c. to reduce image noise
    d. to allow the entire area of interest to be covered during peak contrast enhancement

Answers and Explanations

1. **Answer-b**

2. **Answer-a**

3. **Answer-d**

4. **Answer-a**

5. **Answer-a.** The pyriform sinus of the larynx can be seen distended on a computed tomography (CT) study of the neck if the patient is asked to blow out her cheeks during the scanning process, a modified Valsalva maneuver. Another method of distending the sinus is to ask the patient to pronounce a prolonged "e" sound when scanning.

6. **Answer-a.** Overscans are more common in fourth-generation systems. They are typically performed to reduce the effect of motion.

7. **Answer-b.** Scanning is most commonly performed from the foramen magnum, as the inferior extent of scanning, to the vertex, as the superior extent.

8. **Answer-c**

9. **Answer-a.** Figure 2–2 is from a high-resolution chest CT. This type of study is not performed for metastatic disease because evaluation of the mediastinum is not accomplished. Rather, it is indicated for patients with known diffuse lung disease.

10. **Answer-c.** The dense anatomy of the shoulders creates streak artifacts in the image. Often this can be avoided by instructing the patient to lower his shoulders as much as possible.

11. **Answer-a.** Slice misregistration is caused by the patient's breathing unevenly between scans. Because the number of breath holds is curtailed when using a spiral or cluster technique, the possibility of slice misregistration is reduced.

12. **Answer-a**

13. **Answer-c**

14. **Answer-b.** When image data are used by stacking images to create an image in another plane, the process is called reformation. When raw data are used again to create images, it is referred to as reconstruction. Reconstructions cannot produce images in a different scanning plane.

15. **Answer-a.** When scanning the brain, the entire dose of contrast should be administered before scanning begins. Therefore, the rate at which the contrast is delivered is less critical.

16. **Answer-b.** The identification of normal vascular structures can be difficult if the patient does not possess sufficient mediastinal fat. Intravenous contrast media are indicated in these situations.

17. **Answer-c.** The dorsum sellae supports the pons and carries the abducent nerve in grooves along its lateral aspect.

18. **Answer-c.** Neither Osgood-Schlatter disease nor hemangiomas are malignant in nature. Sarcomas are rarely seen in pediatric patients.

19. **Answer-d**

20. **Answer-c**

21. **Answer-b**

22. **Answer-c.** Anything posterior to the retroperitoneal fascia is considered part of the intra-abdominal compartment, whereas anything lying anterior to this line is in the retroperitoneal compartment.

23. **Answer-c.** "Because the pancreas has essentially the same attenuation coefficient as unopacified bowel and blood vessels, techniques of examination are mainly directed toward identifying all adjacent structures by use of oral and intravenous contrast media."[1]

24. **Answer-d.** The word sinus has been given to two entirely different kinds of spaces connected with the skull. The other type of spaces are the sinuses that are external to the cranium and are hollow spaces, such as the ethmoid and sphenoid sinuses.

25. **Answer-c.** Either the third- or fourth-generation design can be used in a spiral scanner. Some spiral systems include a 1.5- or 2-second tube rotation.

26. **Answer-c.** The bolus phase is often referred to as the arterial phase because contrast has not yet circulated into venous structures. In this phase, it can be difficult to differentiate between low-attenuation liver lesions and venous structures that are not yet opacified.

27. **Answer-a**

28. **Answer-c**

29. **Answer-d**

30. **Answer-b.** The falciform ligament divides the liver into right and left lobes.

31. **Answer-d**

32. **Answer-a.** The brachiocephalic artery is the first vessel off the aortic arch and bifurcates into the right common carotid and the right subclavian arteries. This vessel is often called the innominate artery.

33. **Answer-d.** Biliary passages transport bile from the liver to the hepatic duct, which is then joined by the duct from the gallbladder called the cystic duct; they then form the common bile duct.

34. **Answer-d**

35. **Answer-b**

36. **Answer-a.** To successfully reformat a CT study, all slices must have an identical gantry tilt and image center (i.e., the x and y coordinates must be the same). In addition, they must also have the same display field of view and be contiguous.

37. **Answer-c**

38. **Answer-d**

39. **Answer-c**

40. **Answer-a**

41. **Answer-c**

[1] Federle M, Goldberg H: Abdomen and pelvis. In *Computed Tomography of the Body, with Magnetic Resonance Imaging, 2nd ed, vol 3. Edited by Moss A. Philadelphia, WB Saunders, 1992, p 871.*

42. **Answer-c.** Nonincremental dynamic scanning is often performed to evaluate the enhancement pattern of a lesion. It is commonly used to aid in the diagnosis of liver hemangiomas.

43. **Answer-d.** Respiratory misregistration can result in missing a small lesion caused by a variation in the patient's breathing on successive breath holds. Either spiral or cluster scanning reduces the opportunity of respiratory misregistration by reducing the total number of breath holds required to complete the study.

44. Answer-c

45. Answer-b

46. Answer-c

47. **Answer-a.** Obtaining coronal images is the typical method of scanning the paranasal sinuses. Scanning can be performed with the patient in either the prone or supine position. If the supine position is used, the gantry is angled caudally.

48. Answer-b

49. **Answer-c.** Broadening the window width increases the range of Hounsfield units (HU) that are represented by shades of gray on the image.

50. Answer-c

51. Answer-d

52. Answer-a

53. Answer-b

54. **Answer-c.** Methods of delivering intravenous iodinated contrast medium are still one of the most controversial areas of CT. However, a few areas are universally accepted, such as that body scans should be obtained before the equilibrium phase of contrast enhancement and that the bolus method is the best way to achieve this goal. The timing of contrast media is at least as important as the flow rate in ensuring optimal tissue enhancement. Some researchers suggest that contrast dose can be reduced when using a spiral scan technique, although this is not universally accepted.

55. Answer-b

56. Answer-a

57. Answer-a

58. Answer-c

59. **Answer-b.** A melanoma is a pigmented mole or tumor that may or may not be malignant.

60. **Answer-d.** WORM is the acronym for "write once, read many" and refers to the type of disk that cannot be erased and reused.

61. Answer-d

62. Answer-a

63. Answer-c

64. **Answer-c.** The glabellomeatal line is the imaginary reference line that runs approximately 15° cephalad from the orbital meatal line. The glabella is the surface of the frontal bone lying between the eyebrows.

65. **Answer-d.** A goiter may be caused by a lack of iodine in the diet, thyroiditis, inflammation from infection, a tumor, or hyperfunction or hypofunction of the thyroid gland.

66. **Answer-b**

67. **Answer-a**

68. **Answer-c**

69. **Answer-d.** Aphagia is the inability to swallow; aphonia is the inability to produce speech sound from the larynx (e.g., from chronic laryngitis); and apheresis is the technique used to separate blood into its components.

70. **Answer-d.** Increasing the pitch increases the speed of the table movement relative to the slice thickness and gantry speed. This can be envisioned as pulling the ends of a spring so that each rung is further away from its neighbor. There are no anatomic areas being skipped, although fewer data are being acquired at each location.

71. **Answer-a**

72. **Answer-b**

73. **Answer-b**

74. **Answer-b.** The use of iodinated water-soluble agents varies drastically from that of therapeutic agents in that iodinated agents are given solely for the way they distribute in the body and then are eliminated. Viscosity and high osmolality are the characteristics attributed to the hemodynamic, cardiac, and subjective effects following contrast administration.

75. **Answer-a.** This is an approximate range of normal values. Ranges may vary slightly between laboratories.

76. **Answer-c.** Because of their effects, adrenergics such as Adrenalin are often used to treat iodinated contrast reactions.

77. **Answer-c.** The peak time for the excretion of contrast is approximately 3 minutes following intravenous injection. Peak urine iodine concentration occurs at approximately 60 minutes after injection.

78. **Answer-c.** Reactions are classified into four groups: minor, moderate, major, and fatal. Major reactions require immediate treatment.

79. **Answer-a.** A prothrombin time (PT) is often ordered to evaluate the effects of pharmacological treatment. Based on the results of this laboratory test, dosages of anticoagulant drugs such as heparin and warfarin sodium (Coumadin) can be adjusted.

80. **Answer-b.** Diaphoresis is frequently called a "cold sweat." This important physical sign is determined from visual assessment of the patient.

81. **Answer-c.** Because this wave occurs each time the ventricle contracts, the pulse is an easy and effective way to measure the rate at which the heart is beating.

82. **Answer-b.** A patient's respiratory status is one of four vital signs. Normal is approximately 14 to 20 breaths per minute.

83. **Answer-c.** The range of normal respiratory rates for children is 22 to 28 respirations per minute. In adults, the normal range is 14 to 20 respirations per minute.

84. **Answer-d.** In addition to the rate of the pulse, it is important to note its strength. The descriptive terms usually associated with its strength are: *strong and regular* - good force, even beats; *weak and regular* - poor force, even beats; *irregular* - beats vary between strong and weak within a minute; and *thready* - irregular, weak.

85. **Answer-a.** A blood pressure is taken to monitor a reaction to an intravenous contrast medium or to a systemic drug such as morphine. It is important to know the patient's normal pressure to recognize a sudden deterioration in the patient's condition. Because most inpatients arriving in the CT department have a blood pressure listed in their chart, verification of the listed pressure is adequate.

86. **Answer-d.** Because most finger punctures occur when recapping a syringe, recapping is strongly discouraged. If a needle must be recapped, use the one-hand method: Place the cover on a hard surface and insert the needle into it, without using the other hand.

87. **Answer-c.** Although hand washing seems obvious, it is the rule most frequently ignored in health care settings. To prevent the spread of disease, it is essential that health care workers wash their hands with a liquid or powdered soap after each patient contact.

88. **Answer-b.** Diphenhydramine hydrochloride (Benadryl) is an antihistamine. Drowsiness is by far the most likely side effect from antihistamine use. When higher doses are used, side effects such as dry mouth, stuffy nose, blurred vision, and constipation may also result.

89. **Answer-d.** The precise etiology of iodinated contrast reactions remains unclear. Elevated plasma histamine levels are typical in most anaphylactic reactions but are not a consistent indicator in reaction to contrast media.

Interestingly, increased plasma histamine levels may occur after the infusion of contrast media, but patients do not always exhibit hemodynamic changes or symptoms of anaphylactoid reactions. Conversely, some patients who experience anaphylactoid reactions do not have an associated increase in blood histamines. Although research data suggest that premedication with drugs such as antihistamines and corticosteroids reduces the likelihood of adverse reactions, they cannot be eliminated.

90. **Answer-c.** A solution is referred to as isotonic if it has nearly the same number of particles in solution as water. This property is referred to as a solution's osmolality.

91. **Answer-d.** Osmolality is a characteristic of a solution that describes its number of particles in solution as compared with water. Osmolality is a major component in the side effects that patients experience following the administration of a contrast agent. The biexponential decay curve describes how contrast agents distribute within the plasma. The acute lethal dose (LD_{50}) is the dose required to cause a 50% mortality rate. The ionic nature refers to whether the molecules dissociate in water. Although many contrast agents are nonionic as well as low osmolar, this is not always the case.

92. **Answer-c.** Because most clinical applications of CT involve the use of multiple scans with adjacent or overlapping slices, the dose is calculated by using a routine scan procedure on a Lucite phantom. When the dose is measured and reported, it is known as the multiple scan average dose (MSAD).

93. **Answer-d.** Because of the rotational nature of the x-ray in CT, the center of the patient receives nearly as much radiation as the periphery. This is particularly true of head studies. In conventional radiography, the exit exposure can be as little as 0.1% of the entrance dose. In CT the dose is more uni-

form. Although scatter radiation is much less of a problem in CT than in general radiography, there is still some scatter into the adjacent slices.

94. **Answer-c.** The practice of obtaining written consent from the patient for the administration of intravenous contrast material is not universally accepted. Opponents believe that the process of reading and signing a consent form often increases patient anxiety and increases the likelihood of an adverse reaction. The form offers little protection in cases of litigation. However, consent forms do serve as a reminder to the CT staff to take the time to thoroughly explain the procedure and to answer any questions the patient may have.

95. **Answer-b.** Shaving is not always required for skin preparation and should be done only by the specific order of the physician in charge. The sterile drape is placed *after* the area has been prepared.

96. **Answer-b.** The patient should have only clear liquids for at least 2 hours before scanning to ensure that food in the stomach is not mistaken for a pathological finding. It is important that the patient stay well hydrated to decrease the risk of contrast media–induced acute renal failure (CM-ARF). A patient should never discontinue a prescribed medication without the consent of the referring physician.

97. **Answer-c.** The mortality rate from barium peritonitis is significant. To prevent this condition, a water-soluble solution is recommended whenever there is suspicion of a gastrointestinal tract perforation.

98. **Answer-a.** The drip infusion method relies on gravity to deliver the contrast medium to the patient. The flow rate is altered depending on not only the height of the bottle, but also the intravenous catheter size, the amount of contrast in the bottle, and the viscosity of the contrast material. Therefore, it is impossible to obtain accurate and consistent flow rates with this method. The maximum flow rates available with the drip method are typically only a few milliliters per minute; therefore, peak iodine plasma is never reached and abnormalities may be obscured.

99. **Answer-a.** According to the American Red Cross, check the child's carotid pulse for 5 to 10 seconds before starting cardiopulmonary resuscitation (CPR). It is dangerous to perform chest compressions if the heart is beating. For chest compressions to work, the child must be lying flat on his back on a firm, flat surface with his head on the same level as the heart. A cycle of 5 compressions and 1 breath should be repeated 10 times, then the pulse should be rechecked.

100. **Answer-a.** An adequate size vein is essential if a bolus of contrast is to be delivered. In pediatric patients, this often requires an antecubital site. If an antecubital site is used, the arm should be restrained in extension by attaching an armboard.

101. **Answer-c.** Abortions are typically considered only if the radiation dose exceeds 10 rads.

102. **Answer-d.** This symptom is referred to as cyanosis and is indicative of a breathing problem.

103. **Answer-b.** The bolus phase immediately follows an intravenous bolus injection and is characterized by an attenuation difference of 20 or more HU between the aorta and the inferior vena cava.

104. **Answer-b.** Bleeding is the primary complication of a biopsy procedure. Lesions that are highly vascularized increase this risk. Per-

cutaneous procedures should not be performed on patients with a bleeding disorder. Laboratory tests are performed before the procedure to identify bleeding disorders. Often the patient can be treated with blood products or medications to temporarily remedy the disorder, so that the biopsy can be performed.

105. **Answer-c.** The amount of stress on the tube is directly related to the milliampere (mA) setting and scan time used to perform a study. In spiral scanning, scan time can be as long as 60 seconds. This uninterrupted x-ray output places a heavy burden on the CT tube. In traditional axial scans, there is a brief time for the tube to cool between exposures.

106. **Answer-b.** The term "polychromatic" refers to the fact that an x-ray beam has photons of various intensities. Low-energy photons are often called "soft," whereas the high-energy beams are frequently referred to as "hard." Beam-hardening artifacts result from the preferential absorption of low-energy photons, leaving only the higher-intensity photons to strike the detector array.

107. **Answer-b.** A pixel, or square of data, has two dimensions, width and height. The height is the y axis, and the width is referred to as the x axis.

108. **Answer-d.** Beam attenuation is a basic radiation principle that is illustrated by the fact that higher-density objects absorb (or attenuate) more of the x-ray beam; subsequently, fewer beams reach the photographic film (in conventional x-ray) or the detectors (in CT). The alteration in the beam varies with the density of the structure it passes through. This phenomenon produces images with varying shades of gray.

109. **Answer-c.** Choices b and d both affect beam attenuation capacity, which thereby affects how much x-ray reaches the detector. The

gray scale determines how the Hounsfield values are spread out over the available shades of gray. Although a deficiency in milliampere-seconds (mAs) creates noise in the image, it does not affect the degree of gray in a particular structure.

110. **Answer-a.** HUs are *not* absolute and can be skewed by a variety of factors. Choice c is the definition of a calorie. Adjusting the window setting only changes the way the image is displayed; the Hounsfield measurement remains unchanged.

111. **Answer-b.** The quantity of electrons propelled is typically referred to as tube current and is measured in one thousandth of an ampere, or milliamperes.

112. **Answer-b.** The ability of the tube to rid itself of the heat generated during the production of x-rays is called heat dissipation. This rate is measured in thousand heat units (KHU).

113. **Answer-c.** When a solid-state detector is struck by x-rays, it emits a flash of light. For the computer to use this information, the light must be converted to an electric current. The element in the detector system that makes this conversion is usually a photodiode.

114. **Answer-c.** The digitized data are sent from the reconstruction (often an array-type) processor to the display processor, which then converts it to shades of gray.

115. **Answer-d.** The display processor assigns various HU to each shade of gray in the gray scale. In this way the image can be displayed on the cathode-ray tube (CRT) monitor and subsequently recorded on film.

116. **Answer-d.** Although 120 kilovolt-peak (kVp) is the most common setting used in a clinical CT setting, a variable kVp system allows the operator to increase the setting for examinations on thick, dense parts such as the lumbar spine. Higher kVp settings are also used in the posterior fossa in an effort to reduce beam-hardening artifacts.

117. **Answer-c.** A fourth-generation scanner uses a detector array that is fixed in a 360° circle within the gantry. Second-generation scanners are no longer used. Electron beam imaging is occasionally referred to as the fifth generation of CT scanning. It uses a large electron gun as its x-ray source and is significantly different from other CT designs.

118. **Answer-d.** In this way, a bow tie filter "shapes" the x-ray beam to better fit the study being performed.

119. **Answer-c.** By limiting the amount of x-ray emerging to thin ribbons, collimators directly control the slice thickness. Collimators resemble small shutters with an opening that adjusts to the operator's selection of slice thickness. Because the size of the focal spot affects penumbra, it has a small impact on the sharpness at the edge of the x-ray beam. Neither the matrix size nor the distance between detectors has any effect on slice thickness.

120. **Answer-b.** A wide variety of materials has been used to make solid-state detectors. Manufacturers continually research and upgrade the design of their detectors, often securing patents on the results.

121. **Answer-c.** The process of taking the information from the attenuation profile and projecting it back onto a matrix is called back projection. The disadvantage of back projection is that it produces streaks in the image. To minimize the streaks, a mathematical filtering process called convolution is used before back projection.

122. **Answer-a.** Typically, only a portion of the raw data is used to create the actual image. Changing the display field requires selecting a different portion of the raw data for use in image reconstruction. Image data are used to create multiplanar reformations, three-dimensional models, and to obtain Hounsfield measurements of structures.

123. **Answer-a.** A larger pixel contains information from a larger area of patient anatomy. Spatial resolution is decreased because more data are crammed into each pixel. Each pixel has only one density number, or Hounsfield measurement, which is the average of all the data held in that pixel. If many different densities fall within one pixel, this averaging can obscure the contrariety.

124. **Answer-b.** Ring artifacts are more prevalent in a third-generation system. This is because the same arc of detectors is used repeatedly throughout the scan time. Therefore, if a single detector is defective or misaligned, the result is a ring artifact. In a fourth-generation design, a single faulty detector does not produce a noticeable artifact because many more detectors are used and typically only used once per scan; consequently, bad data are spread evenly across the image.

125. **Answer-d.** All of these factors have an effect on spatial resolution. The display field of view influences the pixel size. The slice thickness determines the extent of volume averaging. The focal spot size controls the penumbra. The modulation transfer function is a measurement of how well the system can process the data in creating an image.

126. **Answer-d.** CT images excel in their low-contrast resolution. For an object to be resolved with standard radiography, there must be at least a 10% difference in object density. In comparison, modern 1024 matrix scanners can resolve a 3–5-mm object having as little as a 0.1% density difference

from the background material. Choice c is evaluated by the mathematical method called the edge response function (ERF). Choice b describes spatial resolution.

127. **Answer-b.** As radiation dose increases, noise decreases because the signal-to-noise ratio increases as more x-ray photons are detected. To double the signal-to-noise ratio, it is necessary to quadruple the mAs.

128. **Answer-a.** Although motion often contributes to air–contrast interface artifacts, they are caused by the notable difference in density between adjacent air and contrast material. These artifacts frequently result from the gastric air–fluid level. Sometimes the artifacts can be reduced by rescanning with the patient in the decubitus or prone position.

129. **Answer-d.** Thinner slices reduce volume averaging by decreasing the amount of patient information included in each voxel.

130. **Answer-b.** In general, wide window widths (400–2000 HU) are best for imaging tissue types that vary greatly. Wider windows encompass greater anatomic diversity, but subtle density discrimination is lost. For this reason, narrow window widths are typically used when imaging the brain, so that the gray matter can be differentiated from the white matter. A wider window width does not eliminate image noise but suppresses the appearance of noise on the image.

131. **Answer-d.** An acute subdural hematoma usually appears as a high-density area that measures from 50–90 HU. Hematoma attenuation values are related to hemoglobin concentration. Clotting removes the lower density components of blood and results in higher attenuation levels. An acute subdural hematoma will be densest in the first three days, gradually decreasing in density during the next 7 to 10 days as the blood elements are broken down.

132. **Answer-a.** On the Hounsfield scale, water is assigned the number 0. Because bone is significantly more dense than water, it possesses a positive CT number.

133. **Answer-d.** The space occupied by the detector plates relative to the surface area of the detector is an aspect of the geometric efficiency of a detector system. The width and spacing of the detectors affect the amount of scatter that is recorded. Simple geometric principles affect this scatter acceptance. Figure 2-13 illustrates this principle.

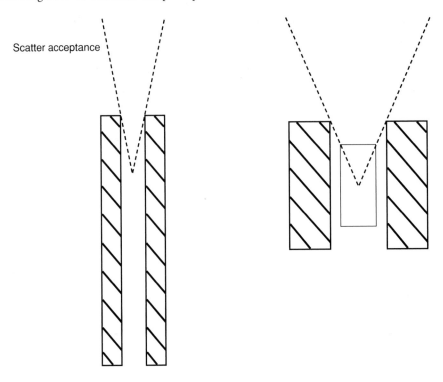

Figure 2-13. Simple geometric principles affect the amount of scatter that reaches the detector.

134. **Answer-c.** The data acquisition system (DAS) is a component of the CT system that is located in the gantry. Its function is to sample each detector cell.

135. **Answer-c.** X-rays are produced when electrons from the filament are rapidly propelled, then suddenly stopped by the target. This process also produces heat.

136. **Answer-a.** The type of optical disk that can be erased and reused is referred to as a magnetic optical disk (MOD). Random access memory (RAM) is temporary memory that stores information when the software is in use. UNIX is a popular operating system that uses the C computer language.

137. **Answer-b.** The size of the generator influences the mAs setting available. Although mAs does not have an effect on CT number accuracy, it affects the level of noise in the image.

138. **Answer-a.** Tungsten, with an atomic number of 74, is often used for target material because it produces a higher-intensity x-ray beam. This is because the intensity of x-ray production is approximately proportional to the atomic number.

139. **Answer-c.** The central processing unit (CPU) is often referred to as the brain of the CT system. It performs mathematical calculations and data comparisons.

140. **Answer-c.** Decreasing the matrix increases the pixel size, thereby decreasing the spatial resolution in the image.

141. **Answer-b.** The CT number is the average of all measurements for that pixel.

142. **Answer-d.** Increasing the pitch can be compared with stretching out a spring. Each rung of the spiral has a more pronounced slant. A mathematical process called interpolation is implemented to minimize the slant so that the image resembles a conventional axial CT image. As the pitch increases, interpolation is less able to adjust for the slant and results in the slice thickness being greater than that selected by the width of the collimator. This increase in the effective slice thickness is sometimes called blooming and is particularly prevalent when pitch is greater than 1.5 (1.5:1).

143. **Answer-b.** Interpolation is a complex statistical method of processing data that examines information from neighboring areas to estimate the missing information. Interpolation is used in all spiral scanners to compensate for the slant.

144. **Answer-c**

145. **Answer-b.** Noise levels for different scanners vary. Fluctuations of CT numbers at varying points in a uniform object indicate noise. Standard deviation, which is the spread of data within a region of interest, can be used to express the degree of noise.

146. **Answer-d.** This quality control test determines if image distortion exists. The distance measured by the CT scanner should match that of the known distance. A difference of 1 mm or less is generally considered acceptable.

147. **Answer-c**

148. **Answer-a.** The spatial resolution improves and the image size enlarges if the raw data are used to reconstruct the data in a larger display field. Simply magnifying the image makes the image larger, but it does not change the pixel size; therefore, the spatial resolution is unchanged.

149. **Answer-c.** Changing the algorithm changes the way the data are projected onto the image matrix. Raw data must be available to accomplish this.

150. **Answer-d.** Protocols for CT angiography often call for a slice thickness of 1 to 3 mm. Adequate contrast enhancement is essential for good results. The pitch is increased to enable the entire area of interest to be scanned.

Exam 3

Questions

1. What is an advantage of scans of the pituitary taken in the coronal plane?

   a. Intravenous contrast material is better visualized.
   b. Streak artifacts are reduced or eliminated.
   c. The patient is more comfortable during scanning.
   d. The patient receives a lower radiation dose.

2. In Figure 3–1 identify the structure indicated by arrow #1.

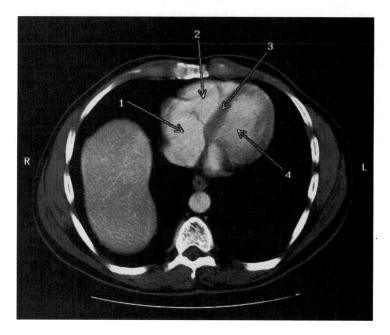

   a. superior vena cava   c. right atrium
   b. right pulmonary artery   d. right ventricle

3. In Figure 3–1 identify the structure indicated by arrow #2.

   a. ascending aorta
   b. left atrium
   c. right atrium
   d. right ventricle

4. In Figure 3–1 identify the structure indicated by arrow #3.

   a. interventricular septum
   b. pericardial fat pad
   c. left ventricle
   d. pericardium

5. In Figure 3–1 identify the structure indicated by arrow #4.

   a. left atrium
   b. left ventricle
   c. left pulmonary artery
   d. descending aorta

6. Which of the following is true concerning computed tomography (CT) studies of the musculoskeletal system?

   a. Intravenous contrast agents are never necessary.
   b. A single bone window is adequate for most studies.
   c. When possible, the normal side should be examined, with the two sides placed symmetrically.
   d. Slice thickness is typically 1–2 mm and never exceeds 3 mm.

7. A typical presentation of an abscess on an iodine enhanced CT study is

   a. that the abscess remains entirely unaffected by the contrast material and presents as a low attenuation area
   b. a low attenuation area surrounded by a ring of enhancement
   c. a high attenuation area because the contrast pools in the abscess, often creating clear fluid levels
   d. that following contrast enhancement, the abscess becomes isodense with the surrounding tissue

8. When is it essential to perform a precontrasted study on the abdomen along with the postcontrasted images?

   a. when the patient has a history of hepatitis B
   b. when the contrasted examination is performed by injection at a high flow rate with the use of a mechanical injector and the scans are performed in a spiral mode
   c. when the entire liver cannot be imaged before the equilibrium phase
   d. when the patient has a history of congestive heart failure

9. Enhancement of most brain lesions is due to

   a. the intrinsic vascularity of the brain
   b. the high subject contrast inherent in the brain
   c. the disruption of the blood–brain barrier
   d. their unique ability to resist intravenous iodinated contrast media

10. Pleural effusion can be defined as

   a. fluid in the pericardial cavity, between the visceral and parietal pericardia
   b. an accumulation of serous fluid in the peritoneal cavity
   c. a local or generalized condition in which the body tissues contain an excessive amount of tissue fluid
   d. the escape of fluid into the thoracic cavity, between the visceral and parietal pleurae

11. What technique can be used to improve visualization of small pituitary lesions?

   a. Intravenous contrast dose is doubled, and scanning begins 45 minutes after injection.
   b. Scans are performed without an intravenous contrast medium.
   c. Intrathecal contrast media is administered by lumbar puncture with scanning approximately 1 hour later.
   d. A bolus of intravenous contrast material is delivered, followed by rapid sequence scanning.

12. In Figure 3–2 identify the structure indicated by arrow #1.

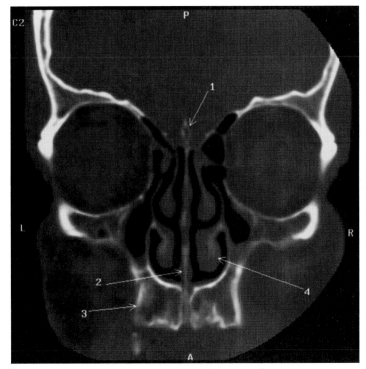

   a. crista galli
   b. inferior nasal turbinate
   c. nasal septum
   d. tuberculum sellae

13. In Figure 3–2 identify the structure indicated by arrow #2.

   a. mandible
   b. hard palate
   c. nasal septum
   d. pterygoid plate

14. In Figure 3–2 identify the structure indicated by arrow #3.

   a. mandible
   b. zygoma
   c. maxilla
   d. greater wing of sphenoid bone

15. In Figure 3–2 identify the structure indicated by arrow #4.

    a. lamina papyracea

    b. hard palate

    c. pterygopalatine fossa

    d. inferior nasal turbinate

16. Which two strategies can reduce the effect of dental fillings in a sinus study?

    a. high milliampere (mA) and short scan time

    b. low kilovolt-peak (kVp) and high-contrast, or bone, algorithm

    c. adjust the angle of the gantry and widen the window width

    d. small focal spot and small display field

17. In filming the brain, why is it common practice to use a wider window width through the posterior fossa?

    a. to reduce the radiation exposure to the patient

    b. to decrease the pixel size

    c. to reduce the appearance of beam-hardening artifacts

    d. to compensate for the small focal spot that is used in the posterior fossa

18. In scanning the brachial plexus, how is the patient positioned on the table?

    a. head first through the gantry, prone, arms up

    b. head first through the gantry, supine, arms down

    c. feet first through the gantry, right decubitus, arms up

    d. feet first through the gantry, prone, arms down

19. In Figure 3–3 identify the structure indicated by arrow #1.

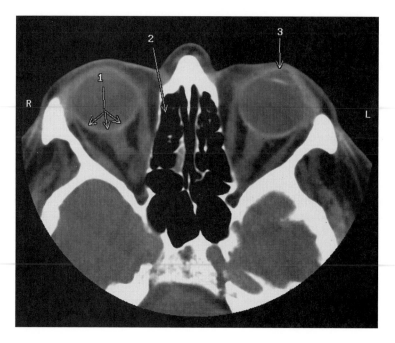

    a. cornea

    b. vitreous humor

    c. optic chiasm

    d. sclera

20. In Figure 3–3 identify the structure indicated by arrow #2.

    a. cavernous sinus

    b. sphenoid sinus

    c. ethmoid sinus

    d. frontal sinus

21. In Figure 3–3 identify the structure indicated by arrow #3.

    a. infundibulum

    b. lens

    c. cornea

    d. retina

22. What are the functions of the preliminary scan that is often referred to as a scout?

    1. ensures that the anatomy of interest falls within the scannable range

    2. determines the optimal mA and scan time for the study

    3. allows the operator to select a start and end location for scans, based on anatomic landmarks

    4. allows slices to be cross-referenced

        a. 1 and 2

        b. 1 and 3

        c. 1, 3, and 4

        d. 1, 2, 3, and 4

23. When a CT protocol includes a scan both before and after the administration of an intravenous contrast agent, all of the following must be done EXCEPT

    a. the contrasted slices should be acquired at the same location as the unenhanced images

    b. an annotation, such as C+, should be included on the enhanced images

    c. the type of contrast material used should be noted on the patient's chart or history form

    d. a consent form should be signed by the patient or their designated agent before the administ ration of an iodinated intravenous agent

24. Which of the following conditions may be visualized in a CT study of the brain?

    a. glioblastoma

    b. Krukenberg tumor

    c. Wilms tumor

    d. plasmacytosis

25. Which of the following is affected by the slice spacing in a CT study?

    a. spatial resolution

    b. quantum mottle

    c. radiation dose to the patient

    d. signal-to-noise ratio

26. In Figure 3–4 identify the structure indicated by arrow #1.

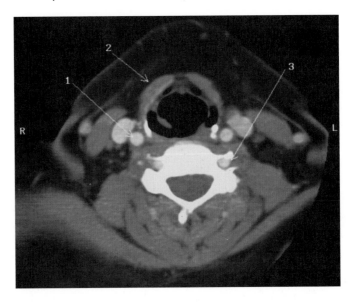

   a. right brachiocephalic vein
   b. right subclavian artery

   c. common carotid artery
   d. external carotid artery

27. In Figure 3–4 identify the structure indicated by arrow #2.

   a. strap muscle
   b. trapezius muscle
   c. epiglottic folds
   d. arytenoid cartilage

28. In Figure 3–4 identify the structure indicated by arrow #3.

   a. internal carotid artery
   b. common carotid artery
   c. vertebral artery
   d. internal jugular vein

29. What is an advantage of using a spiral scan technique for a thorax study?

   a. It is less likely to miss small lesions.
   b. Image noise is decreased.
   c. It is not necessary for the patient to hold her breath.
   d. The software that corrects for table motion also eliminates artifacts from patient movement.

30. What is the name of the pinecone-shaped structure of the brain that can often be seen as calcified in CT images?

   a. choroid plexus
   b. pineal gland
   c. caudate nucleus
   d. middle cerebral artery

31. What is the normal range of CT attenuation measurements for a noncontrasted liver in an adult patient?

   a. −60 to −20 Hounsfield units (HU)
   b. 0 to 25 HU
   c. 38 to 80 HU
   d. 108 to 143 HU

32. What part of the inner ear plays a role in the sense of equilibrium?

   a. incus
   b. epitympanic recess
   c. semicircular canals
   d. superior sagittal sinus

33. In Figure 3–5 identify the structure indicated by arrow #1.

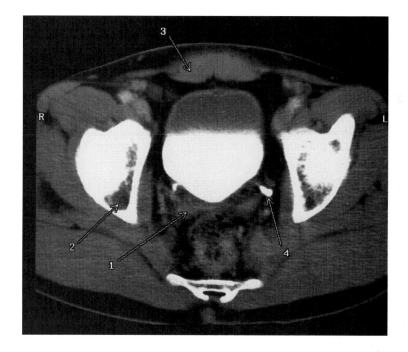

   a. vagina
   b. uterus

   c. seminal vesicle
   d. pyriformis muscle

34. In Figure 3–5 identify the structure indicated by arrow #2.

   a. head of femur
   b. ischium
   c. pubis
   d. iliac wing

35. In Figure 3–5 identify the structure indicated by arrow #3.

   a. rectus muscle
   b. obturator internus muscle
   c. erector spinae muscle
   d. iliacus muscle

36. In Figure 3–5 identify the structure indicated by arrow #4.

    a. spermatic cord
    b. ductus deferens
    c. left ureter
    d. left internal iliac vein

37. By selecting an algorithm, the operator selects

    a. a mathematical formula for processing data
    b. the average photon energy of the x-ray beam
    c. the shades of gray displayed on the image
    d. the center pixel value in the window width

38. What limitation is inherent in using a partial scan to create an image?

    a. Image noise is always excessive because adequate milliampere-seconds (mAs) cannot be achieved.
    b. Scan data cannot be retrospectively segmented.
    c. Longer scan time increases the likelihood of motion artifacts.
    d. Beam-hardening artifacts are increased.

39. The right ventricle sends blood to the

    a. right atrium
    b. left atrium
    c. inferior vena cava
    d. lungs

40. What organ produces the digestive enzymes protease, lipase, and amylase?

    a. gallbladder
    b. stomach
    c. small bowel
    d. pancreas

41. What is being measured in Figure 3–6?

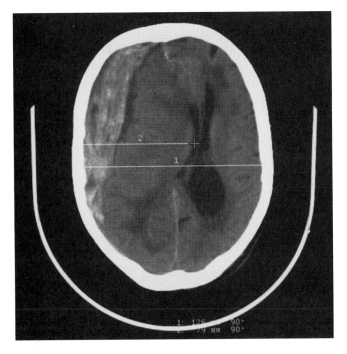

a. the degree of midline shift
b. the degree of ventricular dilatation

c. the density of the abnormality
d. the degree of atrophy

42. What is the most likely diagnosis for the patient in Figure 3–6?

a. severe cerebral atrophy
b. hydrocephalus
c. arachnoiditis
d. subdural hematoma with midline shift

43. The area on the CT image that is defined by the operator and is the first step in most image measurement procedures is called a

a. pixel
b. field of view
c. region of interest
d. scout

44. In a preliminary scout view of a patient, the abdomen is determined to be 300 mm in length. In this CT system, the gantry makes a 360° rotation each second. To cover the entire abdominal area in a single spiral scan, which of the following parameter sets could be selected?

a. 30-second total scan acquisition, 5-mm slice thickness, 1 pitch
b. 30-second total scan acquisition, 5-mm slice thickness, 1.5 pitch
c. 20-second total scan acquisition, 10-mm slice thickness, 1.5 pitch
d. 15-second total scan acquisition, 10-mm slice thickness, 1.5 pitch

45. For a CT study of the abdomen, a drip in-fusion technique delivers 150 ml of contrast. Assuming scanning begins when 100 ml of contrast have been infused, which phase of enhancement does the resulting scans of the liver exhibit?

    a. bolus phase
    b. dynamic phase
    c. nonequilibrium phase
    d. equilibrium phase

46. Of the following studies, which is the most likely to use two different slice thicknesses?

    a. temporal mandibular joints
    b. facial bones
    c. sinuses
    d. cervical spine

47. An area on a scan has an associated measurement of 900 HU. It is most likely composed of

    a. bone
    b. fat
    c. water
    d. air

48. In Figure 3–7 identify the structure indicated by arrow #1.

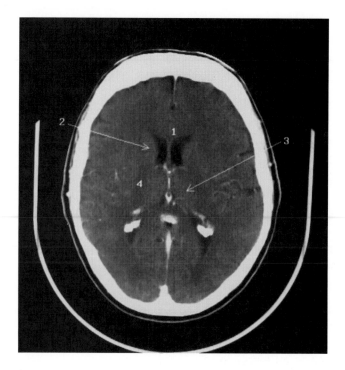

    a. caudate nucleus
    b. corpus callosum
    c. putamen
    d. thalamus

49. In Figure 3–7 identify the structure indicated by arrow #2.

   a. caudate nucleus
   b. internal capsule
   c. hypothalamus
   d. quadrigeminal cistern

50. In Figure 3–7 identify the structure indicated by arrow #3.

   a. globus pallidus
   b. putamen
   c. thalamus
   d. corpus callosum

51. In Figure 3–7 identify the structure indicated by arrow #4.

   a. internal capsule
   b. putamen
   c. thalamus
   d. corpus callosum

52. Crohn disease is primarily a disease of the

   a. gastrointestinal tract
   b. respiratory system
   c. lymphatic system
   d. integumentary system

53. The area within the gantry for which raw data are acquired is called the

   a. scan field of view
   b. display field of view
   c. scannable range
   d. gantry aperture

54. Using image data to create a view in a different imaging plane is called

   a. prospective reconstruction
   b. retrospective reconstruction
   c. back projection
   d. reformation

55. Why would a pelvic study be filmed in a bone window in addition to a soft tissue window?

   a. to reduce artifacts arising from too dense contrast material in the bladder
   b. to better visualize a pelvic malignancy that metastasized to bone
   c. to better visualize the margins of the uterus
   d. to improve the spatial resolution of the image

56. Which of the following has the lowest beam attenuation capacity?

   a. gray matter of the brain
   b. white matter of the brain
   c. liver tissue
   d. vascular structure filled with an iodinated contrast medium

57. Which of the following structures is best visualized with a window width of 2000 and a level set at 350?

   a. lung
   b. liver
   c. gray matter
   d. bone

58. What is the minimum density difference necessary to distinguish abnormal tissue from the surrounding normal tissue?

    a. 3 HU
    b. 10 HU
    c. 20 HU
    d. 50 HU

59. The trachea bifurcates into the

    a. right upper lobe bronchus and left upper lobe bronchus
    b. right interlobar bronchus and left lower lobe bronchus
    c. right main bronchus and left main bronchus
    d. bronchus intermedius and lingular bronchus

60. In Figure 3–8 identify the structure indicated by arrow #1.

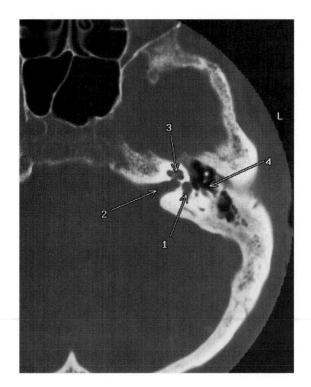

    a. internal jugular vein
    b. cochlea

    c. oval window
    d. facial canal

61. In Figure 3–8 identify the structure indicated by arrow #2.

    a. aditus ad antrum
    b. internal auditory canal
    c. vestibule
    d. mastoid antrum

62. In Figure 3–8 identify the structure indicated by arrow #3.

    a. cochlea
    b. malleus
    c. petrosal nerve canal
    d. aditus ad antrum

63. In Figure 3–8 identify the structure indicated by arrow #4.

    a. mastoid air cells
    b. sigmoid sinus
    c. tympanum
    d. vestibular aqueduct

64. In regard to a three-dimensional CT image, the term disarticulate means

    a. excluding data by reducing the scan field of view
    b. isolating an anatomic part
    c. rotating the three-dimensional image model
    d. separating the image data from the raw data

65. What is the condition that arises when an area of tissue in an organ undergoes necrosis resulting from cessation of its blood supply?

    a. arteriovenous malformation
    b. hemorrhage
    c. infection
    d. infarct

66. A fold of peritoneum that helps attach the liver to the diaphragm is the

    a. falciform ligament
    b. cruciate ligament
    c. azygous vein
    d. papillary muscle

67. What is the name of the eighth cranial nerve that consists of two parts, the vestibular and cochlear nerves?

    a. optic nerve
    b. vagus nerve
    c. acoustic nerve
    d. trigeminal nerve

68. In Figure 3–9 identify the structure indicated by arrow #1.

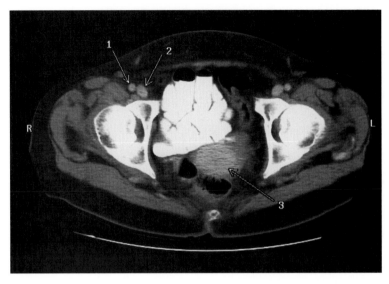

a. femoral vein

b. femoral artery

c. internal iliac vein

d. internal iliac artery

69. In Figure 3–9 identify the structure indicated by arrow #2.

a. femoral vein

b. femoral artery

c. internal iliac vein

d. internal iliac artery

70. In Figure 3–9 identify the structure indicated by arrow #3.

a. urinary bladder

b. vagina

c. prostate gland

d. uterus

71. In a CT study, what effects result from an mAs setting that is too high?

1. higher than necessary radiation dose to the patient

2. loss of contrast in the image

3. increased noise in the image

4. less accurate pixel values

a. 1 only

b. 1 and 2

c. 1, 2, and 4

d. 1, 2, 3, and 4

72. If the gantry in a CT system rotates first in one direction, then stops and rotates in the opposite direction, it

a. is called a rotate–rotate system

b. does not produce spiral scans

c. must be a third-generation system

d. must have solid-state crystal detectors

73. In Figure 3–10 identify the structure indicated by arrow #1.

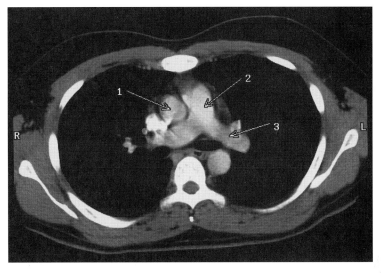

    a. right brachiocephalic vein
    b. right subclavian artery

    c. ascending aorta
    d. superior vena cava

74. In Figure 3–10 identify the structure indicated by arrow #2.

    a. aortic arch
    b. right ventricle
    c. descending aorta
    d. pulmonary trunk

75. In Figure 3–10 identify the structure indicated by arrow #3.

    a. left main bronchus
    b. left pulmonary artery
    c. left atrium
    d. inferior vena cava

76. A partial thromboplastin time (PTT) is often ordered before a CT-guided biopsy. The results are used to

    a. identify deficiencies of coagulation factors, prothrombin and fibrinogen
    b. measure the number of circulating platelets in venous or arterial blood
    c. determine dosages of anticoagulant drugs
    d. determine how long platelets take to work

77. Vicarious excretion is when

    a. contrast material is eliminated from the body through renal excretion
    b. plasma osmolality causes a transfer of water from the blood cells and pulmonary tissue into the plasma space
    c. oral contrast seeps into the peritoneum through a perforation in the gastrointestinal tract
    d. elimination of contrast material occurs through the liver and gut

78. The structural property of a liquid regarding the number of particles in solution compared with water is known as its

    a. ionicity
    b. concentration
    c. salinity
    d. osmolality

79. The laboratory examination typically referred to as a bleeding time is

    a. a measure of the number of circulating platelets in venous or arterial blood
    b. used to determine dosages of anticoagulant drugs
    c. a measure of platelet clot formation after a small puncture wound
    d. a method of measuring blood flow through the pulmonary capillaries using an airtight "body box"

80. What is the normal range of values for a blood urea nitrogen (BUN) test?

    a. 0.7–1.5 mg/dl
    b. 2–5 mg/dl
    c. 10–20 mg/dl
    d. 40–50 mg/dl

81. What is the prevalent symptom experienced by a patient during an acute phase of pulmonary edema?

    a. elevated blood pressure
    b. urticaria
    c. respiratory distress
    d. edema of the ankles

82. The use of iodinated water-soluble agents is based on

    a. their pharmacological action
    b. their therapeutic properties
    c. their distribution in and elimination from the body
    d. the fact that their density is approximately the same as blood

83. Which of the following are considered vital signs?

    1. temperature
    2. pulse rate
    3. respiratory rate
    4. blood pressure
        a. 2 and 4
        b. 3 and 4
        c. 1, 3, and 4
        d. 1, 2, 3, and 4

84. Which of the following are common pulse points?

    a. radial, femoral, and dorsalis pedis
    b. ulnar, iliac, and jugular
    c. digital, antecubital, and popliteal
    d. cephalic, median cubital, and basilic

85. The diastolic figure in a blood pressure recording is a measure of

    a. the pumping action of the heart muscle
    b. the resting phase of the heart
    c. the pulse pressure
    d. the amount of blood pumped out of the heart

86. The pulse rate of children at 5 years of age is

    a. more sporadic than adults
    b. nearly identical to adults
    c. faster than adults
    d. slower than adults

87. Health care workers are at an increased risk for contracting infections. What is the approximate annual number of health care workers infected by the hepatitis B virus?

    a. 200 to 1000 infections, resulting in 50 deaths
    b. 2000 to 3000 infections, resulting in 100 deaths
    c. 8000 to 12,000 infections, resulting in 300 deaths
    d. 18,000 to 22,000 infections, resulting in 650 deaths

88. The complete removal of all organisms and their spores from equipment that is used to perform patient care or procedures is called

    a. universal precautions
    b. medical asepsis
    c. surgical asepsis
    d. body substance precautions

89. What effect do adrenergic agents such as epinephrine (Adrenalin) and dopamine (Intropin) have on the body?

    a. depress the parasympathetic nervous system and act as antispasmodics
    b. relax the walls of blood vessels, permitting a greater flow of blood
    c. prevent the release of histamines into the blood
    d. stimulate the sympathetic nervous system

90. What effect does the administration of chloral hydrate have on a patient?

    a. It depresses and relaxes the central nervous system, thereby reducing mental activity; it is a sedative.
    b. It relaxes the walls of blood vessels, permitting a greater flow of blood; it is a vasodilator.
    c. It prevents or counteracts respiratory depression and other depressive effects of morphine and related drugs; it is a narcotic antagonist.
    d. It depresses the parasympathetic nervous system; it is an anticholinergic.

91. Regarding the identification of a specific reaction caused by contrast administration, asthma-like symptoms without the cutaneous or vascular manifestations are classified as a

    a. vagal reaction
    b. bronchospastic reaction
    c. anaphylactoid reaction
    d. vasomotor effect

92. Which of the following is a true statement concerning iodinated contrast material?

    a. The use of iodinated agents is based on their pharmacological and therapeutic actions.
    b. Abnormal tissue has different contrast enhancement patterns compared with normal tissue; therefore, contrast material is used to increase the difference in density between a lesion and the normal organ parenchyma.
    c. When comparing dose and delivery, contrast agents are not very different from therapeutic agents.
    d. Contrast agents have nearly the same osmolality and viscosity as other intravascular drugs.

93. After the injection of an iodinated contrast medium, patients with brain metastasis have an increased risk of

    a. seizures
    b. dehydration
    c. anaphylactoid reaction
    d. renal failure

94. Which of the following affect the radiation dose to the patient?

    1. scanner generation
    2. collimation
    3. slice spacing
    4. reconstruction filter
      a. 1 and 3
      b. 1, 2, and 3
      c. 2, 3, and 4
      d. 1, 2, 3, and 4

95. Which statement is *true* concerning the multiple scan average dose (MSAD)?

    a. The MSAD can be calculated regardless of the slice spacing.
    b. Scatter radiation is not accounted for in the MSAD.
    c. The MSAD is reported by manufacturers to the United States Food and Drug Administration.
    d. The MSAD is calculated by multiplying the dose from one scan by the number of scans taken.

96. Which of the following sites is best for the injection of an iodinated contrast medium?

    a. peripheral forearm
    b. proximal forearm
    c. hand
    d. central venous line

97. When obtaining a medical history from a patient, it is best to determine whether

    a. there is a family history of iodine allergies
    b. there is a family history of renal failure
    c. the patient has had any previous radiology examinations for which contrast material was administered
    d. the patient has been taking any over-the-counter drugs during the previous week

98. The incidence of allergic response to the oral administration of barium sulfate is quite small. To what is it attributed?

    a. the high osmolality of the solution
    b. barium leaking into the gastrointestinal tract
    c. the high atomic number of barium
    d. additives, such as flavorings, in the suspension

99. When using a central venous catheter for the injection of an iodinated contrast material, which of the following guidelines should be followed?

    1. Use only the distal lumen, which empties into the pulmonary artery.

    2. Flush the line with 10-ml normal saline.

    3. Slow the injection rate to no greater than 0.8 ml/sec.

    4. Do not use any access route that is inflamed.

       a. 1 and 4

       b. 2 and 3

       c. 2, 3, and 4

       d. 1, 2, 3, and 4

100. Which of the following are contraindications to the administration of intravenous contrast material?

    1. asthma

    2. renal failure (unless predialysis)

    3. nephroblastoma

    4. known or suspected pheochromocytoma

       a. 1 and 2

       b. 2 and 4

       c. 1, 3, and 4

       d. 1, 2, 3, and 4

101. All of the following statements are true EXCEPT[1]

    a. cardiopulmonary resuscitation (CPR) must be performed on a firm surface

    b. for CPR to be effective, the head must be level with the heart

    c. bending the elbows during compressions reduces the chance of fracturing a rib

    d. hand contact with the chest should be maintained between each compression

102. In the evaluation of rectosigmoid pathology, which of the following solutions may be administered by enema?

    a. 30 ml of a 1%–3% barium sulfate solution administered 6 hours before scanning

    b. 150–200 ml of a dilute (1%–3%) water-soluble agent administered just before scanning

    c. 600 ml of either a dilute water-soluble or barium sulfate solution administered 60 minutes before scanning

    d. 75–100 ml of a 25% barium sulfate solution administered just before scanning

103. Which of the following is the best way to avoid intravenous contrast extravasation?

    a. Use only low-osmolality contrast media.

    b. Avoid the use of mechanical flow-control injectors.

    c. Use a 21–23-gauge butterfly needle to start the intravenous line.

    d. Monitor the injection site during the initial phase of the injection.

104. Which one of the following examinations delivers the highest patient dose?

    a. postero-anterior (PA) chest x-ray

    b. CT study (body)

    c. barium examination

    d. skull x-ray

[1] The American National Red Cross: *American Red Cross CPR Instructor's Manual*, 1988.

105. When a change in a patient's condition is identified, which of the following should be documented?

    1. date and time
    2. physician involved
    3. method and context of communication
    4. actions taken
        a. 1 and 2
        b. 1 and 4
        c. 2, 3, and 4
        d. 1, 2, 3, and 4

106. The equilibrium phase of contrast enhancement

    a. is the best phase for visualizing hepatic lesions
    b. may never occur in some patients, depending on the diagnosis
    c. requires the contrast media to be administered in a large volume bolus injection
    d. is the worst phase for visualizing hepatic lesions

107. Interpolation, as it is used in CT is

    a. a statistical measure of the spread or dispersion of a set of data, and it is the positive square root of the variance
    b. a mathematical method to estimate a missing value by taking an average of known values at neighboring points
    c. the method used to convert the electric signal to a digital format
    d. the method used to convert light levels into an electric current

108. In CT, the slice thickness may also be referred to as the

    a. latitudinal dimension
    b. transverse dimension
    c. y axis
    d. z axis

109. Another word used to describe a volume element is

    a. pixel
    b. particle
    c. interpolated plane
    d. voxel

110. Structures in a CT image are represented by varying shades of gray. Which one of the following phenomena is responsible for that fact?

    a. beam hardening
    b. Nyquist sampling theorem
    c. beam attenuation
    d. aliasing effect

111. In a CT image, x-ray beams that pass through objects unimpeded are represented by

    a. fewer pixels
    b. a white area on the image
    c. a black area on the image
    d. a long gray scale

112. A CT slice of the abdomen is taken with the following factors: slice thickness = 10 mm, table increment = 10 mm, algorithm = standard, display field of view = 38 cm. The patient is known to have an abdominal lesion with a circumference of 2 mm. The lesion is not seen on the scan series. Which factor is *primarily* responsible?

    a. slice thickness
    b. table increment
    c. algorithm
    d. display field of view

113. In a CT system, why does the anode rotate?

    1. to spread heat over a larger area
    2. to allow increased mAs settings
    3. to prevent pitting in the anode
    4. to reduce the radiation dose to the patient
        a. 1 and 2
        b. 2 and 3
        c. 1, 2, and 3
        d. 1, 2, 3, and 4

114. In what units is the heat dissipation rate of a system listed?

    a. thousand heat units (KHU)
    b. million heat units (MHU)
    c. kilowatts (kW)
    d. mAs

115. Which component of the CT system is responsible for sampling the detector cells?

    a. data acquisition system (DAS)
    b. array processor
    c. photodiode
    d. scintillators

116. The CT process can be broken down into three segments. They are

    a. data acquisition, data retrieval, and data storage
    b. heat production, x-ray production, and image recording
    c. data acquisition, image reconstruction, and image display
    d. beam attenuation, Compton effect, and photoelectric effect

117. What is the power capacity of the CT generator listed in?

    a. kW
    b. kVp
    c. KHU
    d. HU

118. Which of the following is true concerning a CT scanner of a third-generation design?

    a. All spiral, or helical, scanners are of the third-generation design.
    b. Because the tube is closer to the patient, the dose is higher for third-generation scanners, compared with the same technique on a fourth-generation design.
    c. Because the x-ray tube is focused at the bank of detectors, less scatter radiation hits the detectors, compared with the fourth-generation design.
    d. Ring artifacts are much less of a problem with third-generation systems, compared with the fourth-generation design.

119. Which is the *primary* method used to reduce beam-hardening artifacts?

    a. use of filtration to create a more uniform x-ray beam
    b. increasing mA
    c. use of a rotating target
    d. regular system calibrations

120. Which of the following are characteristics of solid-state detectors?

    1. low efficiency
    2. sensitive to temperature and moisture
    3. may exhibit afterglow
    4. also called scintillators
        a. 1 and 2
        b. 1 and 3
        c. 2, 3, and 4
        d. 1, 2, 3, and 4

121. Why is it necessary to apply a filter function to an attenuation profile (convolution)?

    a. to minimize streaks
    b. to increase the signal-to-noise ratio
    c. to eliminate ring artifacts
    d. to reduce radiation exposure to the patient

122. A lumbar spine is scanned using a 48-cm scan field of view. The display field has been adjusted so that the spine lies in the center of the image (x = 0, y = −5). Which of the following diagrams depicts how the raw data are collected?

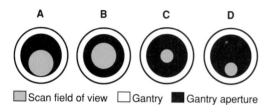

☐ Scan field of view ☐ Gantry ■ Gantry aperture

123. A partial scan can be defined as

    a. a scan in which two matching samples are taken 180° apart
    b. a scan taken from a tube arc of 180° plus the degree of arc of the fan angle
    c. a scan taken from a tube arc of 3608 plus the width of the field of view
    d. a scan that has been aborted after more than half of the data has been collected

124. Why is a fourth-generation CT system sometimes referred to as a rotate only scanner?

    a. Only the tube rotates, the detectors remain fixed in a 360° ring.
    b. The tube continues to rotate in the same direction.
    c. The tube and detector rotate in unison, facing opposite one another.
    d. The tube and detector each rotate in the opposite direction.

125. A graphical representation of the CT system's capability of passing information through it to the observer is called

    a. interpolation
    b. modulation transfer function (MTF)
    c. receiver–operator characteristics
    d. contrast–detail response

126. In CT the size of the object visible on an image depends on

    a. the level of contrast inherent in the object
    b. the type of detector
    c. Ohm's law
    d. the electron-binding energy

127. Which of the following reduce the visibility of noise?

    1. Display the image using a wide window width.
    2. Display the image with a large field of view.
    3. Use a high-contrast, or bone, algorithm.
    4. Use a smoothing algorithm.
        a. 1 only
        b. 1 and 4
        c. 2 and 3
        d. 1, 2, and 3

128. What system assigns a given number of HU to each level of gray in the CT image?

    a. histogram
    b. gray scale
    c. image compression
    d. back projection

129. The window width of a specific CT image is set at 300, and the level (or center) is set at 100. How is a structure with a measurement of 280 HU displayed?

    a. It is white.
    b. It is a light shade of gray.
    c. It is a dark shade of gray.
    d. It is black.

130. The fraction of photons removed from the beam, per centimeter, in an absorber is often referred to as

    a. attenuation coefficient
    b. contrast transfer function
    c. MTF
    d. MSAD

131. Which factors produce an image with the best spatial resolution?

    a. 128 matrix and a small focal spot
    b. 256 matrix and a large focal spot
    c. 512 matrix and a large focal spot
    d. 1024 matrix and a small focal spot

132. The detector spacing is

    a. the distance from the wall of one detector to the closest wall of the neighboring detector
    b. the distance between the walls of a single detector (the detector opening)
    c. the distance from the center of one detector to the center of the adjacent detector
    d. the depth of the detector

133. The ability of the detector to capture transmitted photons and change them to electronic signals is called

    a. geometric efficiency
    b. detector efficiency
    c. linear attenuation coefficient
    d. photon proficiency

134. How can out-of-field artifacts be avoided?

    a. calibrate according to manufacturer's recommendations
    b. ensure that enough samples are taken by using a full, rather than a partial, scan
    c. select the appropriate scan field of view
    d. select the appropriate kVp setting

135. What is a disadvantage of high mA settings?

    a. More stress to the x-ray tube is caused by the heat generated.
    b. Smaller focal spot must be used.
    c. It may produce ring artifacts.
    d. Beam-hardening artifacts increase.

136. What is the function of analog-to-digital converters?

    a. They translate the raw data onto a matrix.
    b. They convert the light levels from a solid-state detector into an electric current.
    c. They convert electric signals into a digital format.
    d. They take digitized data and translate it into shades of gray.

137. When CT is compared with film/screen radiography

    1. the radiation dose to the patient is much less in CT
    2. the low-contrast detectability is superior in CT
    3. the spatial resolution is worse in CT
    4. superior digital data storage options are available with CT

    a. 1 and 2
    b. 1 and 3
    c. 2, 3, and 4
    d. 1, 2, 3, and 4

138. Which of the following artifacts may appear in a CT image?

 1. cupping
 2. aliasing
 3. phase encoding
 4. truncation
    a. 1 and 2
    b. 1 and 3
    c. 1, 3, and 4
    d. 1, 2, 3, and 4

139. An increase in the kVp increases the

 a. image noise
 b. maximum x-ray energy
 c. spatial resolution
 d. scatter radiation

140. What is the function of the photodiode in a solid-state detector system?

 a. ionizes the gas in the chamber to produce an electric current
 b. converts the light level into an electric current
 c. attenuates some of the x-ray photons while allowing other photons to pass through to the detector unimpeded, relating to the density of the anatomic structure
 d. accelerates the ions by the high voltage on the detector plates

141. "The number of collimator widths covered in one gantry rotation"[2] describes

 a. interpolation
 b. standard deviation
 c. pitch
 d. attenuation coefficient

142. For which application are the raw data necessary?

 a. to create a three-dimensional model
 b. to decrease the display field size
 c. to create a histogram
 d. to obtain a Hounsfield measurement of a specific structure

143. An aliasing effect artifact may occur when

 a. a partial scan is used
 b. a detector malfunctions
 c. an overscan is used
 d. an x-ray tube is worn

144. A magnification factor of 1.5 is used to enlarge the image data, resulting in

 a. a decrease in the pixel size
 b. an increase in the pixel size
 c. an inaccuracy in any subsequent distance measurement
 d. an image that allows more accurate cursor placement for measurements

145. The most significant way to suppress quantum noise in the CT image is to increase the

 a. matrix size
 b. scan field of view
 c. x-ray photons
 d. target–detector distance

146. A 20-cm water phantom is scanned, and five regions of interest are placed within the resulting image. The maximum deviation of a CT number at the center and the periphery of the image indicates the degree of

 a. spatial resolution
 b. contrast resolution
 c. linearity
 d. cross-field uniformity

[2] Fishman E, Jeffrey B: *Spiral CT: Principles, Techniques, and Clinical Applications.* New York, Raven Press, 1995, p 4.

147. What is the process of using image data to create a view in a different body plane called?

    a. retrospective reconstruction
    b. prospective reconstruction
    c. reformation
    d. multiplanar histogram

148. What is necessary to create a three-dimensional model?

    a. Raw data must be available.
    b. All slices must be contiguous.
    c. Original images must be scanned with a higher mAs setting.
    d. Original images must be scanned with the widest slice thickness available.

149. In CT image creation using a third-generation design, a complete set of ray sums is known as a

    a. star network
    b. topogram
    c. spatial frequency filter
    d. view

150. The process of applying a filter function to an attenuation profile is known as

    a. back projection
    b. convolution
    c. archiving
    d. reformation

Answers and Explanations

1. Answer-b. Although the pituitary gland is most often scanned in both the axial and coronal planes, use of the latter provides more useful information. Streak artifacts from the dense bone of the sella turcica are common in the axial plane and are reduced or eliminated in the coronal plane.

2. Answer-c

3. Answer-d

4. Answer-a

5. Answer-b

6. Answer-c. Because the anatomy of the musculoskeletal system varies from one region to another, the specific factors used are tailored to the examination. In nearly all cases, it is important to film the images in both a soft tissue and bone window. Iodinated contrast may be helpful when evaluating tumors and their relation to other structures. Although an 8–10-mm slice thickness is adequate for most parts, small structures may require thinner slices.

7. Answer-b

8. Answer-c. Metastatic lesions may fill in and become the same density as surrounding tissue in the equilibrium phase of contrast enhancement. Therefore, if scans cannot be obtained before this phase because of limitations concerning the speed of the computed tomography (CT) system, then a pre-contrasted study should be performed.

9. Answer-c. Because the enhancement of most brain lesions results from disruption of the blood–brain barrier and not from vascularity of the lesion, it is important to administer the entire dose of intravenous contrast before scanning.

10. Answer-d

11. Answer-d. Because pituitary lesions are in an area without a blood–brain barrier, a bolus technique may improve visualization.

12. Answer-a

13. Answer-c

14. Answer-c

15. Answer-d

16. Answer-c. A less commonly used third option is reconstructing the raw data with a soft, or low-contrast, algorithm.

17. Answer-c. Because of the dense bone of the cranium, beam hardening is particularly prevalent in the posterior fossa. Window settings are applied to an image after it has been reconstructed; therefore, it cannot affect the radiation dose or the pixel size. Even if a small focal spot is used, no change in window setting is required.

18. Answer-b

19. Answer-d

20. Answer-c

21. Answer-c

22. Answer-c

23. Answer-d. The use of consent forms for contrast agent administration is not universally accepted.

24. Answer-a. A glioma is a sarcoma of neuroglial origin. A glioblastoma is a neoplasm of the central nervous system, particularly the cerebrum. Glioma retinae is a malignant tumor of the retina that occurs in children.

25. Answer-c. Slice spacing affects whether slices are contiguous, gapped, or overlapping. Compared with slices taken in a contiguous fashion, gapped slices decrease the patient's total radiation dose whereas overlapping slices increase the patient's total exposure.

26. Answer-c

27. Answer-a

28. Answer-c

29. Answer-a. Because many or all slices can be taken within a single patient breath hold, misregistration is reduced or eliminated using a spiral scan technique. In addition, the data can be retrospectively reconstructed in an overlapping fashion. This technique may visualize a lesion that was not distinguishable because its data straddled two slices and, therefore, was averaged in with normal tissue. Retrospectively changing the data incrementation allows all of the data from a lesion to appear in a single slice.

30. Answer-b. The pineal gland got its name from its pinecone shape. It can frequently be identified as a calcified structure on a CT image.

31. Answer-c. Attenuations lower than this range often indicate fatty infiltrate of the liver.

32. Answer-c

33. Answer-c

34. Answer-b

35. Answer-a

36. Answer-c

37. Answer-a. By selecting a specific algorithm, the operator can influence how data are filtered in the back projection process. Some algorithms create a higher contrast image by enhancing the difference between adjacent structures, whereas other algorithms create a "smoother" image by suppressing the difference.

38. Answer-b. On many CT systems, the raw data for an image can be segmented and an image produced by eliminating one of the segments. Segmenting is done to eliminate motion that occurred in only a portion of the scan time. Segmenting is not possible, however, if a partial scan was used to create the original image.

39. Answer-d. The ventricles are considerably larger and thicker walled than the atria because they carry a heavier pumping burden. The right ventricle sends blood to the lungs, whereas the left ventricle pumps blood to the rest of the body.

40. **Answer-d**

41. **Answer-a**

42. **Answer-d**

43. **Answer-c.** The region of interest may be circular, square, elliptic, rectangular, or it may be custom drawn by the operator.

44. **Answer-c.** Using the following formula to calculate the area of anatomy covered in a spiral scan,

$$\text{Total acquisition time} \times \frac{1}{\text{Rotation time}}$$

$$\times \text{Slice thickness} \times \text{Pitch}$$

$$= \text{Amount of anatomy covered}$$

and using the parameters from choice c

20-second acquisition time

$$\times \frac{1}{\text{1-second rotation time}}$$

$$\times \text{10-mm slice thickness}$$

$$\times \text{1.5 pitch}$$

$$= \text{300-mm anatomy covered}$$

Choices a, b, and d would cover 150 mm, 225 mm, and 225 mm, respectively.

45. **Answer-d.** The last phase of tissue enhancement is the equilibrium phase. The attenuation difference between the aorta and the inferior vena cava is less than 10 Hounsfield units (HU). This is considered the worst stage for visualization of hepatic tumors.

46. **Answer-c.** A common protocol for scanning the sinuses is coronal images produced with a 3-mm slice thickness through the osteomeatal complex and a 5-mm slice thickness throughout the rest of the study.

47. **Answer-a**

48. **Answer-b**

49. **Answer-a**

50. **Answer-c**

51. **Answer-a**

52. **Answer-a**

53. **Answer-a.** The scan field of view is a circle that lies in the absolute center of the gantry. Raw data are collected for anything that falls within the circle. The display field is another circle, which can be smaller than the scan field circle, that determines what part of the raw data is displayed on the image. The gantry aperture refers to the size of the gantry opening, and the scannable range is the portion of the CT table that can be scanned.

54. **Answer-d.** Reformatting is often confused with reconstruction, but the two terms are very different. Reformatting requires only image data, whereas reconstruction is accomplished with raw data.

55. **Answer-b**

56. **Answer-b.** The attenuation capacity of a structure is directly related to its density.

57. **Answer-d.** Wider window widths, such as those used to display bone, encompass greater anatomic diversity, but subtle density discrimination is lost.

58. **Answer-b.** Often iodinated contrast media is used to create or enhance the density difference between adjacent structures.

59. **Answer-c**

60. **Answer-c**

61. **Answer-b**

62. **Answer-a**

63. **Answer-c**

64. **Answer-b.** Three-dimensional imaging offers the technologist the ability to create diagnostic images unobtainable with other imaging modalities. A specific bone or vessel can be isolated and viewed, thus preventing nearby structures from obscuring crucial information.

65. **Answer-d.** Infarcts may result from occlusion or stenosis of the supplying artery or, more rarely, from occlusion of the vein that drains the tissue.

66. **Answer-a.** The falciform ligament is a wide fold of peritoneum that is attached to the inferior surface of the diaphragm, the internal surface of the right rectus muscle, and the convex surface of the liver.

67. **Answer-c**

68. **Answer-b**

69. **Answer-a**

70. **Answer-d**

71. **Answer-a.** In contrast to conventional radiography, an overexposed CT image is not degraded.

72. **Answer-b.** To produce spiral scans, the gantry must rotate continuously in the same direction, which is accomplished by using a slip-ring device in the gantry. Both the terms rotate–rotate and third generation refer to systems in which the detector array rotates in conjunction with the tube.

73. **Answer-c**

74. **Answer-d**

75. **Answer-b**

76. **Answer-a.** A partial thromboplastin time (PTT) is a complex method for testing the normalcy of the coagulation process. A normal range is 24 to 36 seconds. A prolonged time indicates deficiencies of a coagulation factor. A PTT is not diagnostic for platelet disorders.

77. **Answer-d.** Although the elimination of contrast media from the body is primarily by renal clearance, in the case of complete cessation of renal function, elimination of the contrast medium is through the liver and gut. This is called vicarious excretion.

78. **Answer-d.** Both the terms "ionic" and "osmolality" refer to a contrast agent's chemical composition. However, ionic refers to whether the particles dissociate in water, whereas the term osmolality refers to how many particles are in solution compared with water.

79. **Answer-c.** Knowledge about the length of bleeding time is essential to have before most surgeries or even extensive dental extractions. Because the primary complication of CT-guided biopsy is excessive bleeding, it is often part of the prebiopsy work-up.

80. **Answer-a.** This is an approximate range of normal values. Ranges may vary slightly between laboratories.

81. **Answer-c.** Pulmonary edema is the effusion of fluid into air vesicles and into the interstitial tissue of the lungs. Symptoms are extreme dyspnea; rapid, labored breathing; cough with frothy, bloodstained expectoration; cyanosis; and cold extremities.

82. **Answer-c.** Iodinated contrast agent administration varies dramatically from other intravenous pharmaceuticals. Intravenous contrast agents are used because of the way they disburse and then are eliminated from the body.

83. **Answer-d.** All four procedures are used for assessment and are collectively referred to as vital signs.

84. **Answer-a.** A pulse can only be taken by depressing an artery, not a vein. Figure 3–12 shows the common pulse points.

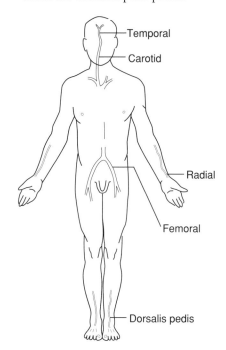

Figure 3-12. Common pulse points.

85. **Answer-b.** The blood pressure consists of two numbers: the systolic pressure written over the diastolic pressure. (To remember the placement of these values, think *d*iastolic = *d*own). The diastolic pressure is the lowest pressure in the vessel. It occurs between heart beats when the heart is at rest. Pulse pressure is the difference between the two measurements.

86. **Answer-c.** The normal pulse rate for a 5-year-old child is approximately 95 beats per minute, whereas a 1-year-old child typically has a pulse rate of 110 beats per minute. In adults the normal range is 70 to 80 beats per minute.

87. **Answer-c.** Occupationally contracted infections pose a threat to health care workers. The Occupational Safety and Health Administration (OSHA) requires health care employers to provide hepatitis B immunization to employees, at employer expense. It also requires a written plan that outlines actions employees should take when possible exposure takes place.

88. **Answer-c.** Surgical asepsis requires the removal of all organisms, whereas medical asepsis is a method of reducing, but probably not eliminating, the number of pathogenic microorganisms. Surgical aseptic techniques are required whenever the skin is to be punctured.

89. **Answer-d.** Adrenergic agents stimulate the sympathetic nervous system, thereby causing a constriction of the blood vessels, an increase in cardiac output, an increase in blood pressure, and relaxation of the smooth muscle lining of the respiratory tract.

90. **Answer-a.** Chloral hydrate (Noctec, Aquachloral) is sometimes used as a sedative for children or other patients who are anxious about the CT examination. It is used because it does not depress respirations or the cough reflex. As with all medication, dosage should be carefully checked with a physician before administration.

91. **Answer-b.** The first step in the treatment of an adverse reaction to contrast media is the proper identification of specific symptoms. A reaction that is manifested by wheezing but is not accompanied by facial edema is a bronchospastic reaction. These are typically treated by the administration of oxygen and a β_2 agonist such as metaproterenol (Alupent), terbutaline (Brethaire), or albuterol (Proventil) delivered by a single-use metered dose inhaler.

92. **Answer-b.** The statements in choices a, c, and d are untrue. Iodinated agents are used for their method of distribution in and elimination from the body. There is an enormous difference in dose and delivery from therapeutic agents. It is typical that therapeutic agents are given in very small quantities at regular intervals, whereas contrast medium dose is often large and given very rapidly. Although most intravascular agents are isotonic, contrast material can have up to seven times the osmolality of body fluids, and their viscosity is much greater.

93. **Answer-a.** Patients who have diseases that affect the blood–brain barrier may be at increased risk from contrast administration because the contrast material may enter the brain more readily. In the general population, seizures after intravenous contrast medium administration are rare, with an incidence of approximately 0.01%. However, patients with brain metastasis have a post-contrast seizure rate of 6% to 19%.[1]

94. **Answer-b.** The reconstruction filter or algorithm does not affect patient radiation dose and can be changed retrospectively, provided raw data are still available. Fourth-generation scan geometry places the tube closer to the patient; so with the same technique the dose is higher. Collimators reduce radiation by curtailing scatter radiation. Slice spacing that allows overlapping slices increases the radiation dose, whereas a slice spacing that leaves unradiated gaps between slices decreases the radiation dose.

95. **Answer-a.** The multiple scan average dose (MSAD) is calculated by scanning a Lucite phantom in a manner that mimics a typical scanning procedure. Contiguous, overlapping, or gapped scan protocols can be used. By taking a series of CT slices, the effects of scatter radiation are accounted for in the measurement. The CT dose index (CTDI) is performed only with contiguous slices and is reported to the United States Food and Drug Administration by scanner manufacturers.

96. **Answer-b.** A medially placed antecubital vein or the proximal forearm are the best sites for administration of contrast material. The use of peripheral forearm or hand veins must be carefully monitored, and injection rates lowered. Indwelling central lines are not recommended for contrast injection because many have a lower pounds per square inch (psi) rating than standard intravenous catheters.

97. **Answer-c.** If a patient has had a previous adverse reaction to iodinated contrast material, special consideration must be taken before the patient is given contrast a second time. Because patients may not recognize the term "iodinated contrast material," it is best to incorporate the many aliases into the question. For example, "Have you ever had an examination where they used iodine? It is sometimes called contrast medium or x-ray dye."

[1] Katzberg R: *The Contrast Media Manual.* Baltimore, Williams & Wilkins, 1992, p 16.

98. **Answer-d.** Barium sulfate is an inert substance that passes through the body basically unchanged. Allergic reactions are rare; approximately 1 in 500,000 cases are generally attributed to the additives in the suspension.

99. **Answer-c.** The lumen that accesses the pulmonary artery should never be used for the injection of contrast media because of the risk of introducing a pulmonary embolus. The proximal or venous infusion port (VIP) lumina can be used because these access the right atrium. The injection rate should be lowered because many indwelling central lines have a lower psi rating than standard intravenous catheters. Flushing the line with saline assesses its patency.

100. **Answer-b.** There is disagreement about which conditions should be considered absolute contraindications to intravenous iodinated contrast media. It is universally accepted that patients with renal failure should be given contrast media only if they undergo dialysis shortly following its administration. Iodinated contrast media can incite a hypertensive crisis in patients with pheochromocytoma. Another accepted contraindication is a previous major reaction to contrast media. Special evaluation should be given to patients who have sickle-cell anemia (active crisis is a contraindication) or multiple myeloma.

101. **Answer-c.** The American Red Cross recommends keeping the elbows straight when performing compressions.

102. **Answer-b.** In order for contrast material given orally to reach the rectosigmoid colon, a minimum of 600 ml must be given 6 to 12 hours before scanning. If oral contrast does not opacify the rectosigmoid colon, 150 to 200 ml of a 1%–3% water-soluble agent can be administered by enema.

103. **Answer-d.** The injection site should be monitored, at least during its initial phase; if swelling is detected, the injection should be immediately stopped. Although low-osmolality contrast media are less injurious to soft tissue than are high-osmolality agents, the incidence of extravasation remains unchanged. Intravenous catheters, such as Angiocaths, are recommended for contrast injection. When proper precautions are followed, mechanical flow-control injectors are safe and effective.

104. **Answer-b.** The highest source of man-made radiation exposure, aside from radiation therapy, results from diagnostic procedures. CT is the highest contributor. The typical effective dose equivalent values for the listed procedures are: postero-anterior (PA) chest x-ray = 1–5 mrem, CT study (body) = 500–1500 mrem, barium examination = 300–800 mrem, skull x-ray = 10–20 mrem.[2]

105. **Answer-d.** In addition, the instructions received from the physician and the response of the patient should be documented.

106. **Answer-d.** The equilibrium phase is considered the worst phase for lesion detection, particularly lesions of the liver. In some cases scanning in this phase may be inferior to an unenhanced study. The equilibrium phase is the last phase and is characterized by a difference of less than 10 HU between the aorta and the inferior vena cava.

107. **Answer-b.** This method is used in spiral scanning. The system takes the slanted spiral data and estimates what its appearance would be if the slices were taken axially, with each slice parallel to the others. The greater the slant (i.e., the higher the pitch), the more interpolation required. Choice a is the definition for standard deviation.

[2] Huda W, Slone R: *Review of Radiologic Physics.* Baltimore, Williams & Wilkins, 1995, pp 139–140.

108. Answer-d. Data that form a CT slice are sectioned into elements. Each element has three dimensions (as does the patient). The width of the section is the x axis, and the height is the y axis. The length is referred to as the z axis, which is the depth or longitudinal plane that corresponds with the head to foot direction of the patient lying on a CT table. This data segmentation is illustrated in Figure 3–13.

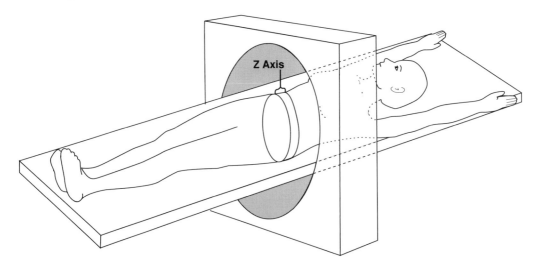

Figure 3-13. The Z axis corresponds to the head-to-foot direction of the patient and is defined by slice thickness.

109. Answer-d. A volume element is a unit of data in the shape of a cube. It is often called a voxel.

110. Answer-c. Beam attenuation is a basic radiation principle that is illustrated by the fact that higher-density objects absorb (or attenuate) more of the x-ray beam, resulting in fewer x-ray photons reaching the photographic film (in conventional x-ray) or the detector (in CT). The amount of x-ray that reaches the detector is reflective of the densities within the patient and is represented by varying shades of gray.

111. Answer-c. By convention established from general radiography, x-ray beams that pass through objects unimpeded are represented by a black area on the image. Conversely, x-ray beams that are completely stopped by an object cannot be detected; therefore, the place on the image where the beam is halted is white. All intermediate attenuations are represented by various shades of gray.

112. Answer-a. Volume averaging, or partial volume effect, is most likely responsible for nonvisualization of the lesion. Because the slice thickness is set at 10 mm in this scenario, data from a 2-mm lesion are being averaged with the data from 8 mm of normal tissue. The result can be an image that "hides" the lesion.

113. Answer-c. When electrons strike the target material, x-ray and heat are produced. Heat is a negative result because it can damage the anode. Therefore, the target rotates to spread the heat over a larger area, preventing damage such as pitting and allowing higher techniques.

114. Answer-a

115. Answer-a. The data acquisition system (DAS) samples the detector cells as many as 1000 times per second.

116. **Answer-c.** The steps of CT image creation can be broadly categorized into getting the data (data acquisition), using the data (image reconstruction), and showing the data (image display).

117. **Answer-a.** Generator ratings are listed in kilowatts (kW). Kilovolt-peak (kVp) refers to the voltage used to propel electrons from cathode to anode. Heat dissipation is measured in thousand heat units (KHU); HU is a measure of beam attenuation.

118. **Answer-c.** Because, in the third-generation design, the x-ray source remains focused directly on the detector bank and both detector array and tube rotate opposite one another, very little scatter radiation strikes the detector. Scatter radiation is more problematic in the fourth-generation design because the x-ray source rotates within a stationary ring of detectors. Because of the placement of tube and detectors, it is not possible to focus the source directly on the detector, and more scatter reaches the detector. This concept is illustrated by Figure 3–14.

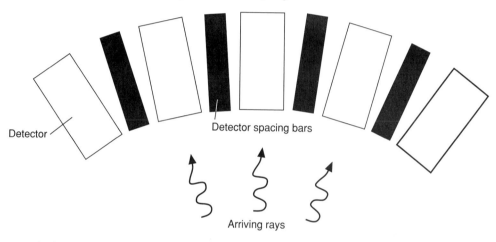

Figure 3-14. Third-generation systems allow the x-ray tube to be focused directly on the detector bank, which reduces the amount of scatter that reaches the detectors.

119. **Answer-a.** Filtration is used to create a more uniform x-ray beam, thereby reducing beam-hardening artifacts.

120. **Answer-c.** The primary advantage of a solid-state detector system is its ability to sense the x-ray photons that strike it. This property is referred to as its efficiency. As a rule, they tend to be less stable than xenon gas detectors. Some solid-state detectors, particularly the older ones, have problems with afterglow. Because the solid-state detectors give off a brief flash of light when struck by an x-ray photon, they are often referred to as scintillators.

121. **Answer-a.** Streaks are inherent in the back projection process; therefore, it is essential to apply a mathematical filtering process before back projection.

122. **Answer-b.** By selecting a 48-cm scan field of view, the operator acquires data in a circular shape, with a diameter of 48 cm lying in the absolute center, or isocenter, of the gantry. The display field selects how much data are to be used to create the image; in this situation 15 cm of data are used. The centering, or x and y, coordinates select the segment of data to be used. In this case $x = 0$, so the image is centered in the horizontal direction, and $y = -5$, so the displayed image center is lower than the raw data center.

123. Answer-b. Because the tube travels only 180° in a partial scan, only one set of samples are taken. This type of scan must be selected before the start of scanning; simply aborting a full scan more than half way through data acquisition does not produce an image and cannot be referred to as a partial scan. A full scan is taken from a tube arc of 360°, with two matching samples acquired 180° apart. A scan taken from a tube arc of 360° plus the width of the field of view is referred to as an overscan.

124. Answer-a. In a fourth-generation design, the detectors remain fixed and only the tube rotates in a circular path. Whether the tube first rotates in one direction, then stops to rotate in the opposite direction, instead of rotating continually in the same direction is not dependent on generation, but rather on whether the system contains a slip-ring device.

125. Answer-b. The modulation transfer function (MTF) is a measure of the capability of the scanner to produce an image that accurately reflects the object scanned. It offers information on the resolution capability of the scanner as a function of spatial resolution. The MTF is often represented by a graph such as the one in Figure 3–15.

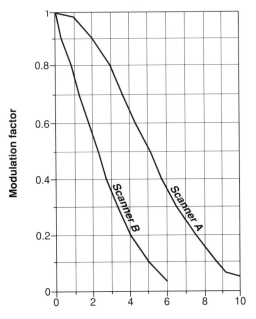

Spatial frequency (line pairs per cm)

Figure 3-15. Classic MTF graph.

126. Answer-a. The size of the object that is visible on an image depends on the level of contrast in the object. A smaller object is visible if the object's density varies dramatically from its surroundings (e.g., a small calcified nodule in a lung field). Other factors that affect the size of the visible object are image noise and the window setting at which the image is displayed.

127. Answer-b. Smoothing algorithms reduce the visibility of noise by averaging each pixel with its neighbor. A high-contrast, or bone, algorithm amplifies the appearance of noise. Wide window widths also help disguise noise. Display field has no effect on noise.

128. **Answer-b.** Although there are more than 4000 possible HU, the cathode-ray tube (CRT) monitor can display only 256 shades of gray. More limiting still is the fact that the human eye can only differentiate approximately 20 shades of gray. To compensate for these limitations, the gray scale is used. This system assigns a given number of HU to each level of gray in the CT image. If a wide range of HU is to be displayed on one image (i.e., a wide window width), then many HUs are assigned to each shade of gray. The inverse is also true; a narrow window width results in each shade of gray being assigned just a few HU.

129. **Answer-a.** The window width selects the range of HU that is to be represented as shades of gray on the image. The window level determines which, of all the possible HU, are to be included. In this example, the total HU to be represented is 300. Because the center is set at 100, the HU depicted are −50 to 250. This is calculated by dividing 300 in half, then subtracting the dividend from the center (100) to find the lower limit. Add the dividend to 100 to find the upper limit. Everything that falls below these numbers appears black, whereas everything above appears white. Figure 3–16 depicts this process.

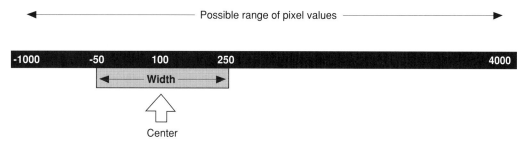

Figure 3-16. The window width selects the range of Hounsfield values displayed. The window level selects the center value.

130. **Answer-a.** As x-ray photons travel through an object, some of the x-ray energy passes through although some is stopped or scattered. This phenomenon is referred to as attenuation of the x-ray beam. The attenuation coefficient is a number derived from a specific strength beam as it travels through a specific substance. For example, with a CT scanner that is operating in the typical range of 120 kVp, the linear attenuation coefficient for water is approximately 0.19 cm^{-1}. This means that when the beam passes through 0.1 cm of water, about 1.9% of the photons are either absorbed or scattered.

131. **Answer-d.** The matrix size is inversely proportional to the pixel size. A smaller pixel reduces the amount of volume averaging in the image. A small focal spot reduces the penumbra. The penumbra affects the amount of blur in the image. Both volume averaging and blur negatively affect the spatial resolution in an image.

132. **Answer-c.** Detector spacing is determined by measuring the distance from the center of one detector to the center of the neighboring detector. The distance between the walls of a single detector is referred to as the detector aperture, as shown in Figure 3–17.

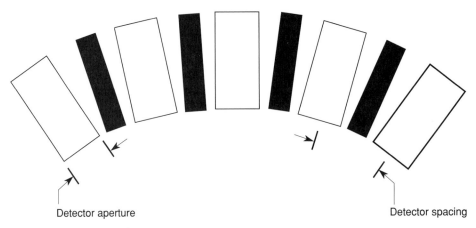

Detector aperture   Detector spacing

Figure 3-17. Detector spacing and aperture.

133. **Answer-b.** Solid-state detectors have a higher rate of discerning photons that strike them as compared with xenon gas detectors. This is because xenon gas must be kept in chambers, and the chamber absorbs some of the x-rays so they do not reach the detector.

134. **Answer-c.** Most manufacturers recommend using a scan field of view that just encompasses the patient. If too small a scan field is selected with these systems, out-of-field artifacts may result. Some systems have incorporated corrections within the software so that the incorrect scan field does not produce these artifacts. An example of a system with this type of software compensation is the Picker PQ-2000. In any case, it is important to follow manufacturer's guidelines concerning field size.

135. **Answer-a.** If all other factors are kept constant, increasing the milliampere (mA) setting reduces image noise. However, the increase places a greater cooling burden on the tube. mA has no bearing on ring artifacts.

136. **Answer-c.** Raw data from the detector are in the form of an electric current. It must be converted into a digital format to be used by the computer. Analog-to-digital converters carry out this function.

137. **Answer-c.** The patient radiation dose is substantially higher in CT than for film/screen studies of the same body part.

138. **Answer-a.** Cupping artifacts are a type of artifact that result from beam hardening. Aliasing effects are seen when there are not enough samples taken, as is sometimes the case when a partial scan is used. Both phase encoding and truncation artifacts appear only in magnetic resonance (MR) images.

139. **Answer-b.** The kVp affects the speed that the electrons strike the target and, therefore, affects the maximum x-ray photon energy produced.

140. **Answer-b.** In a solid-state detector system, the x-ray photons strike the detector material, which in turn emits a brief flash of light. This process is often called scintillation, and the material that emits the light when struck

is referred to as a scintillator. The light must be converted to an electric current for use as raw data. This conversion is accomplished by the photodiode.

141. **Answer-c.** Pitch is a term most commonly used in spiral scanning. It describes the relationship between table speed, slice thickness, and gantry rotation. For example, if the pitch is described as 1^3 and the slice thickness is set at 5 mm, the table moves at a speed that allows the gantry to rotate once every 5 mm of table travel.

142. **Answer-b.** Changing the display field requires the raw data. In doing this, the pixel size decreases and the spatial resolution increases.

143. **Answer-a.** Aliasing effect artifacts are characterized by fine streaks and are caused by too few samples. Because a partial scan obtains information from only 180° plus the degree of arc of the fan angle, fewer samples are used in image formation and artifacts may result.

144. **Answer-d.** Image magnification is not synonymous to changing the display field size. Because magnification uses only image data and not raw data, pixel size is not affected. A magnified image retains accuracy in all image measurements.

145. **Answer-c.** The most significant way to suppress noise in the image is to increase the x-ray photons by increasing the milliampere-seconds (mAs). This results in a higher radiation dose to the patient.

146. **Answer-d.** Ideally, an image produced from an object that has only one density should have a constant CT number, regardless of where the region of interest is placed within the image. Cross-field uniformity is a method of assessing this function of a CT system. A phantom is scanned, and five regions of interest are placed within the resulting image. The maximum CT number deviation should be no greater than 2 HU.

147. **Answer-c.** The reformation process can be compared with stacking up slices of bread so that they resemble an intact loaf and proceeding to cut the loaf in a different fashion. Only the image data are used for this function. Reconstruction is the process of creating an image from raw data.

148. **Answer-b.** As in multiplanar reformations, all images must share the same display field, center, gantry tilt, and table height; and all images must be contiguous. Three-dimensional models are created from image data only. It is not necessary to increase technique on the original study to produce acceptable three-dimensional images. Although any slice thickness can be used, a general rule is that the thinner the slice, the better the three-dimensional model.

149. **Answer-d.** A view in the CT process can be compared with observing an object from a single angle. It takes many views to obtain a true understanding of the shape of the object. Similarly, it takes many views to create the CT image.

150. **Answer-b.** Different mathematical functions can be used to enhance or suppress parts of the data. Depending on the manufacturer, the filter function used may be called algorithm, convolution filter, kernel, or CR filters.

---

[3] Pitch also may be described as a ratio of table speed to slice thickness. A pitch of 1 would be written as the ratio 1:1.

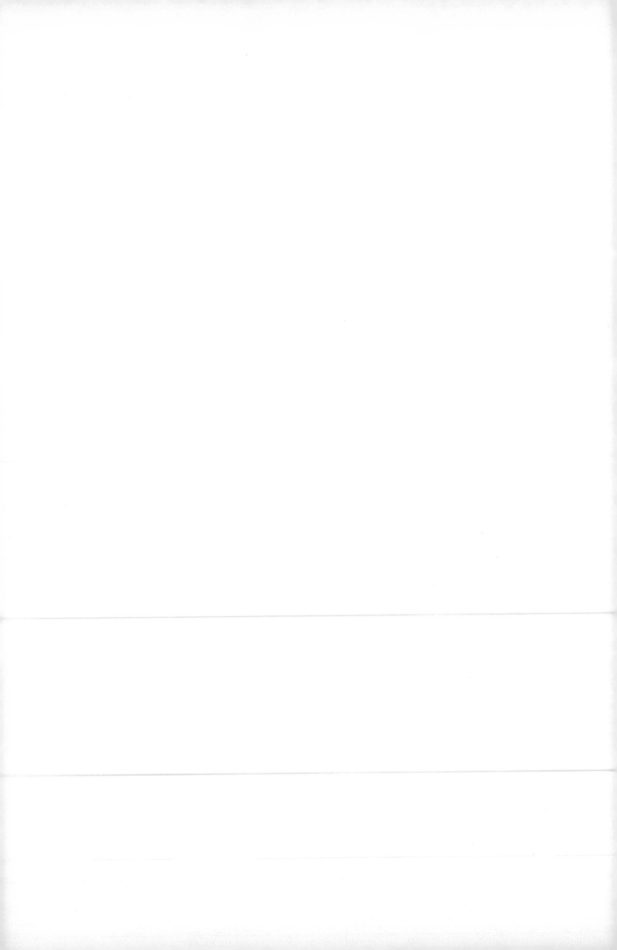

Exam 4

Questions

1. All of the following are associated with computed tomography (CT) findings of a cerebral infarction EXCEPT

   a. edema is often seen initially

   b. swelling may obliterate adjacent sulci

   c. a low-density change often extends to the cortical surface and obliterates the normal gray–white distinction

   d. if scans are performed with iodinated contrast, within six hours of onset, the infarct becomes brightly enhanced

2. In Figure 4–1 identify the structure indicated by arrow #1.

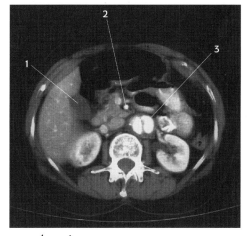

   a. hepatic cyst

   b. pancreatic cyst

   c. gallbladder

   d. ascending colon (unopacified)

3. In Figure 4–1 identify the structure indicated by arrow #2.

   a. ampulla of the duodenum

   b. splenic vein

   c. superior mesenteric vein

   d. left gastric artery

4. In Figure 4–1 identify the structure indicated by arrow #3.

   a. renal arteries

   b. aortic dissection

   c. aortic valve

   d. common iliac arteries

5. Selecting a 5-mm slice thickness with a 5-mm table increment, rather than a 10-mm slice thickness with a 10-mm table increment, to perform an examination of the abdomen

   a. increases the partial volume effect

   b. increases the likelihood of detecting small lesions

   c. decreases the patient's total radiation exposure

   d. decreases the tube cooling time between scans

6. Most brain lesions are enhanced with the administration of intravenous contrast media due to the disruption of the blood–brain barrier. Which of the following is an exception to that rule?

   a. metastatic lesion of the brain

   b. primary cancer tumor of the brain

   c. meningioma

   d. tumor of the pituitary gland

7. The thin, delicate middle membrane that encloses the brain and spinal cord is called the

   a. arachnoid membrane

   b. dura mater

   c. pia mater

   d. encephalon

8. Which diagnosis requires raw data to be reused to reconstruct images in a bone (high-contrast) algorithm?

   a. acoustic neuroma
   b. herniated lumbar disk
   c. dissecting thoracic aneurysm
   d. arteriovenous malformation

9. A CT examination of the paranasal sinus often incorporates two different slice thicknesses. The thinner slices are used to

   a. evaluate acoustic neuromas
   b. differentiate chronic sinusitis from a common cold
   c. assess an abscess of the sphenoid sinus
   d. evaluate the osteomeatal complex

10. All of the following are options for performing a CT examination of the neck EXCEPT

   a. hyperextension of the patient's neck
   b. a spiral scan technique
   c. patient is asked to perform a modified Valsalva maneuver
   d. patient is asked to pronounce a prolonged "e" during scanning

11. Which of the following is true concerning the use of intravenous iodinated contrast medium for CT studies of the thorax?

   a. It is universally accepted that routine chest studies be performed with intravenous contrast media.
   b. When spiral scanning is used, scan acquisition and contrast administration should begin together.
   c. Many experts believe that when performing an examination of the thorax, intravenous contrast is not necessary under ordinary circumstances and should be used only in specific instances.
   d. A biphasic injection technique should never be used when scanning the thorax.

12. A teratoma can be described as

   a. a congenital tumor containing one or more of the three primary embryonic germ layers; therefore, hair and teeth as well as endodermal elements may be present
   b. a congenital endocrine disorder caused by failure of the ovaries to respond to pituitary hormone stimulation
   c. carcinoma of the fatty tissue
   d. a malignancy of the skin that rarely metastasizes

13. In Figure 4–2, arrow **#1** depicts

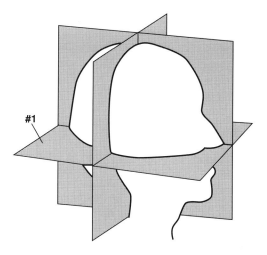

a. a coronal plane   c. a sagittal plane
b. a central plane   d. an axial plane

14. Which of the following techniques improves the quality of a multiplanar reformation?

    a. Scan using a wide slice thickness.
    b. Select 140 kilovolt-peak (kVp) for scanning.
    c. Acquire scans with a slice spacing that is less than the slice thickness.
    d. Use a long scan time (5 seconds or longer).

15. In a study that includes scans taken both before and after contrast enhancement, why should the slices be taken at identical table positions?

    a. to facilitate comparisons between unenhanced and enhanced images
    b. to reduce the partial volume effect
    c. to reduce the radiation exposure to the patient
    d. to increase the number of samples per view, thereby improving spatial resolution

16. What is the advantage of using the glabellomeatal line rather than the orbital meatal line when scanning the brain?

    a. Visualization of contrast media within the middle cerebral artery is improved.
    b. Fewer slices are required to complete the study.
    c. A wider slice thickness can be used.
    d. Radiation exposure to the lens of the eye is reduced.

17. In Figure 4–3 identify the structure indicated by arrow #1.

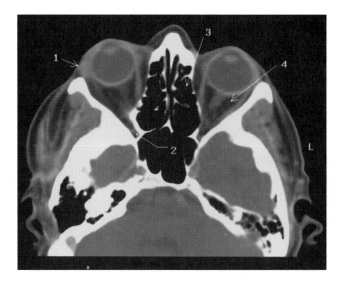

a. cornea
b. lens

c. lateral rectus muscle
d. lacrimal gland

18. In Figure 4–3 identify the structure indicated by arrow #2.

a. foramen ovale
b. optic canal
c. optic chiasm
d. check ligament

19. In Figure 4–3 identify the structure indicated by arrow #3.

a. ethmoid sinus
b. sphenoid sinus
c. frontal sinus
d. maxillary sinus

20. In Figure 4–3 identify the structure indicated by arrow #4.

a. lateral rectus muscle
b. orbital fat
c. sclera
d. vitreous humor

21. Which of the following is a common practice when performing a high-resolution chest protocol?

a. 10-mm slice thickness
b. contiguous slices
c. rapid scan acquisition following a large bolus of contrast media
d. filming each lung field separately using a small field size

22. Which modifications are possible when a new spiral scanning system replaces an older CT system?

1. The contrast dose can be reduced.
2. Precontrast scans of the liver can be eliminated.
3. The use of a mechanical flow-control injector can be discontinued.
4. Time allotted each patient can be reduced.

a. 1 and 4
b. 3 and 4
c. 1, 2, and 4
d. 1, 2, 3, and 4

23. Ninety percent of pheochromocytomas are located in the

    a. adrenal glands
    b. kidneys
    c. pancreas
    d. bladder

24. Fatty infiltrate of the liver may result from

    a. chemotherapy
    b. intravenous iodinated contrast media
    c. stress
    d. chronically elevated blood cholesterol levels

25. The upper part of the brain stem that serves as a pathway between the cord and other parts of the brain is the

    a. corpus callosum
    b. superior sagittal sinus
    c. pons
    d. falx cerebri

26. Why do incorrect milliampere-second (mAs) settings affect CT images differently than incorrect mAs settings in conventional radiography?

    a. X-ray energy is substantially higher in CT.
    b. X-ray energy is substantially lower in CT.
    c. The detectors have a large dynamic range compared with that of film/screen radiography.
    d. Cross-sectional images require a much lower radiation dose to produce.

27. Which of the following factors should be adjusted when slice thickness is decreased from 10 to 3 mm?

    a. Increase display field.
    b. Decrease matrix size.
    c. Double window level.
    d. Increase mAs.

28. Assume an acceptable axial study is taken using the following technique: scan time = 2 seconds, milliamperes (mA) = 150, kVp = 120, slice thickness = 5 mm, slice spacing = 5mm. The study is to be repeated using a spiral scanning technique in which the tube rotates 360° each second. To produce a comparable study, which of the following adjustments should be made?

    a. 2:1 pitch
    b. 1.5 pitch
    c. 300 mA
    d. 10-mm slice thickness with 50% retrospective data overlap

29. What vein is formed by the superior and inferior mesenteric veins and the splenic vein?

    a. celiac axis
    b. common hepatic vein
    c. portal vein
    d. gastric vein

30. What is being measured in Figure 4–4?

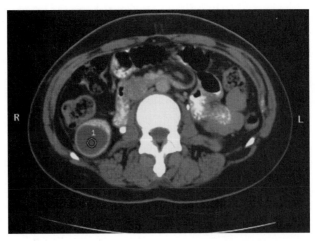

a. gallbladder

b. abscess of colon

c. malignant renal mass

d. benign renal cyst

31. Which bone of the cranium resembles a bat with its wings outstretched and legs extended downward posteriorly?

a. ethmoid

b. maxilla

c. sphenoid

d. temporal

32. The adenohypophysis and the neurohypophysis make up the

a. thyroid gland

b. pituitary gland

c. adrenal gland

d. salivary glands

33. In a spiral scan of the abdomen, the following parameters have been selected: total scan acquisition time = 20 seconds, slice thickness = 7 mm, pitch = 1, tube arc = 1 second for each 360° rotation. It is determined that the area of interest cannot be fully covered with the above parameters, and the scan is at least 60 mm too short. Of the following, which adjustment might be made to allow the entire area to be scanned in this single spiral acquisition?

1. Increase slice thickness to 10 mm.

2. Increase pitch to 1.5.

3. Slow the tube arc to 1.5 seconds for each 360°.

4. Increase the total scan acquisition time to 29 seconds.

    a. 1 only

    b. either 1 or 3

    c. either 2 or 4

    d. 1, 2, or 4

34. What is an advantage of using CT to guide percutaneous procedures?

    a. The needle can be viewed when it is being inserted.
    b. A much smaller needle can be used under CT guidance, reducing associated risks.
    c. CT images provide precise localization of lesions, and the exact tip of the needle within the structure can be visualized.
    d. The procedure is less expensive as compared with biopsies performed with ultrasound or fluoroscopy guidance.

35. In Figure 4–5 identify the structure indicated by arrow #1.

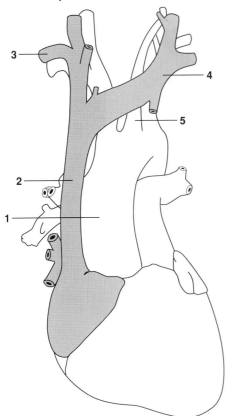

    a. superior vena cava
    b. ascending aorta
    c. descending aorta
    d. pulmonary trunk

36. In Figure 4–5 identify the structure indicated by arrow #2.

    a. superior vena cava
    b. ascending aorta
    c. right subclavian vein
    d. right common carotid artery

37. In Figure 4–5 identify the structure indicated by arrow #3.

    a. superior vena cava
    b. right brachiocephalic vein
    c. right subclavian vein
    d. right internal jugular vein

38. In Figure 4–5 identify the structure indicated by arrow #4.

    a. superior vena cava
    b. aortic arch
    c. left common carotid artery
    d. left brachiocephalic vein

39. In Figure 4–5 identify the structure indicated by arrow #5.

    a. brachiocephalic artery
    b. left subclavian artery
    c. left pulmonary artery
    d. left common carotid artery

40. Which of the following may be a reason for overlapping slices in a CT study?

    1. reduces the radiation exposure to the patient
    2. reduces beam-hardening artifacts
    3. places more slices within a specific area of interest
    4. improves the quality of multiplanar reformations

    a. 3 only
    b. 3 and 4
    c. 2, 3, and 4
    d. 1, 2, 3, and 4

41. A lipoma is composed of what type of tissue?

    a. connective tissue
    b. bone
    c. fat
    d. muscle

42. Which of the following window settings is best to evaluate emphysema?

    a. window width 1800, window center −600
    b. window width 600, window center 1800
    c. window width 350, window center 50
    d. window width −600, window center 1600

43. In Figure 4–6 identify the structure indicated by arrow #1.

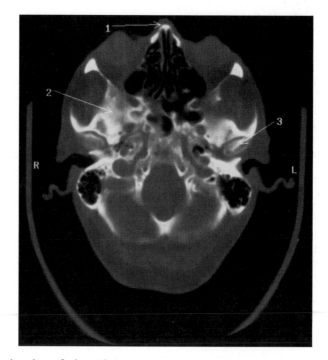

    a. perpendicular plate of ethmoid sinus
    b. nasal bone

    c. zygoma
    d. vomer

44. In Figure 4–6 identify the structure indicated by arrow #2.

    a. greater wing of sphenoid bone
    b. maxilla
    c. zygoma
    d. petrous bone

45. In Figure 4–6 identify the structure indicated by arrow #3.

    a. mandibular condyle
    b. petrous bone
    c. foramen ovale
    d. body of sphenoid bone

46. The vein of Galen is located in which body part?

   a. brain
   b. neck
   c. thorax
   d. abdomen

47. What technique can be used to differentiate the margins of the pancreas from the duodenum?

   a. water-soluble contrast medium administered by enema
   b. place the patient in a right decubitus position
   c. place the patient in a left decubitus position
   d. scan approximately 2 hours after the patient ingests 600 ml of an oral contrast medium

48. In Figure 4–7 identify the structure indicated by arrow #1.

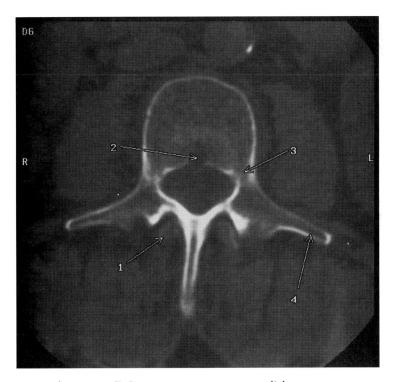

   a. superior articular process (L3)
   b. inferior articular process (L2)

   c. pedicle
   d. lamina

49. In Figure 4–7 identify the structure indicated by arrow #2.

   a. nerve root
   b. anterior longitudinal ligament
   c. basivertebral vein
   d. ligamentum flavum

50. In Figure 4–7 identify the structure indicated by arrow #3.

   a. lamina
   b. pedicle
   c. superior articular process
   d. transverse process

51. In Figure 4–7 identify the structure indicated by arrow #4.

   a. transverse process
   b. spinous process
   c. annulus fibrosus
   d. articular facet

52. What is the most superior part of the sternum?

   a. xiphoid process
   b. manubrium
   c. ensiform
   d. gladiolus

53. What is an advantage of reconstructing raw data and altering the incrementation?

   a. decreases the radiation dose to the patient
   b. allows the operator to change to a smaller focal spot
   c. reduces the slice thickness
   d. may decrease the partial volume effect

54. In Figure 4–8 identify the structure indicated by arrow #1.

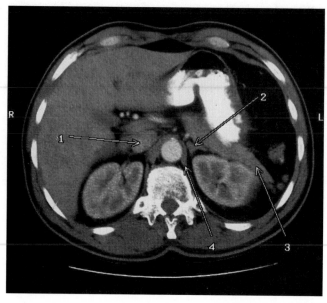

   a. portal vein
   b. pancreatic head

   c. celiac axis
   d. inferior vena cava

55. In Figure 4–8 identify the structure indicated by arrow **#**2.

 a. left adrenal gland

 b. splenic artery

 c. superior mesenteric vein

 d. left renal vein

56. In Figure 4–8 identify the structure indicated by arrow **#**3.

 a. pancreatic head

 b. pancreatic tail

 c. uncinate process of pancreas

 d. jejunum

57. In Figure 4–8 identify the structure indicated by arrow **#**4.

 a. vertebral artery

 b. superior mesenteric vein

 c. falciform ligament

 d. diaphragmatic crus

58. Of the following, which injection technique was most likely used to create Figure 4–8?

 a. rapid bolus injection, scanning started 30 seconds after start of injection

 b. rapid bolus injection, scanning started 3 minutes after start of injection

 c. drip infusion, scanning started 30 seconds after start of infusion

 d. drip infusion, scanning started after 50 ml of contrast was infused

59. In addition to providing a greater radiation dose to the patient, what detrimental effect does increasing the mAs produce?

 a. increases the heat load on the x-ray tube

 b. increases the image noise

 c. increases beam-hardening artifacts in the image

 d. decreases contrast resolution in the image

60. What display function allows areas on consecutive cross-sectional images to be traced and their outline then superimposed over the scout image?

 a. correlate

 b. histogram

 c. dual window

 d. coronal reformation

61. The ridgelike lateral walls of the entrance to the larynx are the

 a. palmate folds

 b. aryepiglottic folds

 c. circular folds

 d. vestigial folds

62. In Figure 4–9 identify the structure indicated by arrow #1.

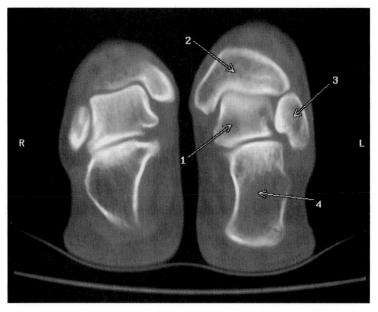

   a. talus   c. calcaneus

   b. cuboid   d. media cuneiform

63. In Figure 4–9 identify the structure indicated by arrow #2.

   a. fibula

   b. navicular

   c. tibia

   d. cuboid

64. In Figure 4–9 identify the structure indicated by arrow #3.

   a. tibia

   b. lateral cuneiform

   c. fifth metatarsal

   d. lateral malleolus of fibula

65. In Figure 4–9 identify the structure indicated by arrow #4.

   a. calcaneus

   b. talus

   c. cuboid

   d. navicular

66. Including a bone window on a CT study of the brain helps to visualize

   a. intercranial bleeds

   b. arteriovenous malformation

   c. skull fractures

   d. hydrocephalus

67. What is necessary to perform stereotactic surgical planning in conjunction with CT imaging?

   a. a CT system that allows histogram measurements

   b. a surgical suite

   c. a special localizing device that is placed on the CT scanning table

   d. a CT system that has spiral capabilities

68. In Figure 4–10 identify the structure indicated by arrow #1.

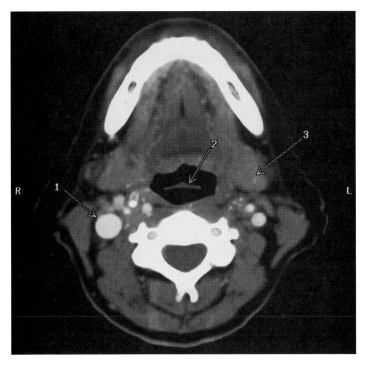

    a. internal carotid artery   c. parotid gland
    b. internal jugular vein   d. common carotid artery

69. In Figure 4–10 identify the structure indicated by arrow #2.

    a. larynx
    b. arytenoid cartilage
    c. esophagus
    d. epiglottis

70. In Figure 4–10 identify the structure indicated by arrow #3.

    a. submandibular gland
    b. parotid gland
    c. tongue
    d. middle scalene muscle

71. The large veins of the cranial cavity that are formed by the dura mater are called

    a. arterioles
    b. venules
    c. fissures
    d. sinuses

72. The left subclavian artery is

    a. the first vessel arising from the aortic arch
    b. a branch of the superior mesenteric artery
    c. the third vessel arising from the aortic arch
    d. divided further into the right and left carotid arteries

73. The tenth cranial nerve has both motor and sensory functions. It has a wider distribution than any of the other cranial nerves. What is it called?

    a. glossopharyngeal nerve

    b. accessory nerve

    c. vagus nerve

    d. abducent nerve

74. In Figure 4–11 identify the structure indicated by arrow #1.

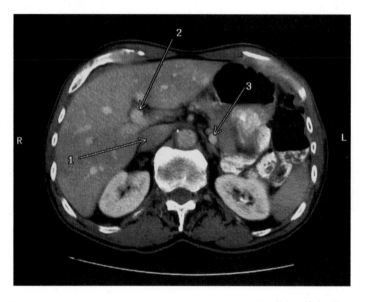

    a. portal vein   c. caudate lobe of the liver

    b. duodenum   d. inferior vena cava

75. In Figure 4–11 identify the structure indicated by arrow #2.

    a. portal vein

    b. gallbladder

    c. celiac artery

    d. common bile duct

76. In Figure 4–11 identify the structure indicated by arrow #3.

    a. superior mesenteric vein

    b. superior mesenteric artery

    c. portal vein

    d. common bile duct

77. An air embolus is

    a. a protein molecule that is essential to the immune system and is produced in response to bacteria, viruses, or other foreign substances

    b. necrosis of tissue, caused by decreased blood flow

    c. a stationary blood clot in a vessel

    d. a rare but life-threatening complication that occurs when a large amount of air enters a vein

78. Why is it recommended to warm contrast media before intravenous injection?

    a. Heating increases the osmolality of the contrast agent, therefore reducing vasodilatation, heat, pain, and hemodynamic effects.

    b. As temperature increases, the volume of solution decreases, and the milligrams of iodine per milliliter (mgI/ml) increases significantly.

    c. Heating the contrast medium to body temperature decreases the viscosity and facilitates rapid injection.

    d. The temperature of the contrast agent is directly proportional to its density; therefore, warming increases density, which increases the contrast's beam attenuation capabilities.

79. Contrast reactions that are accompanied by a temporary drop in blood pressure, bronchospasms, facial edema, urticaria, and laryngeal edema are generally classified as

    a. minor reactions
    b. moderate reactions
    c. major reactions
    d. fatal reactions

80. Which units are used to report prothrombin time (PT)?

    a. cubic millimeters (mm³)
    b. seconds
    c. minutes
    d. hours

81. What is always necessary before procedures that involve puncture or incision of the skin?

    a. Laboratory values for blood urea nitrogen (BUN) and creatinine are drawn, and the results deemed within normal limits.

    b. Hair is removed.

    c. A physician must be readily accessible.

    d. Skin preparation includes thorough cleansing, followed by application of an antiseptic solution.

82. Bradycardia can result from

    a. excitement or exertion
    b. athletic training
    c. loss of blood
    d. amphetamines

83. Under what circumstances would a carotid pulse be preferable to a radial pulse?

    a. whenever a more accurate pulse reading is needed

    b. if the patient has been diagnosed with a carotid stenosis

    c. if the radial pulse is difficult to count or is weak

    d. if the patient has lymphoma

84. Which of the following describes a patient in shock or with significant blood loss?

    a. marked increase in pulse rate and rapid, shallow breathing

    b. sudden decrease in pulse rate and a sudden elevation in blood pressure

    c. very rosy skin color and rapid increase in body temperature

    d. slurred speech and a sudden decrease in body temperature

85. In general, an average diastolic pressure less than 50 mm Hg may indicate

    a. hypertension
    b. shock
    c. hypoxemia
    d. cardiac arrest

86. Which of the following is a general principle concerning cleaning?

    a. Always clean from the least contaminated area toward the most contaminated area.
    b. Always clean from the most contaminated area toward the least contaminated area.
    c. Always clean from the bottom up.
    d. Only those pieces of equipment that have come in contact with a body substance require cleaning.

87. Which one of the following statements is true concerning antihistamines such as diphenhydramine hydrochloride?

    a. Antihistamines are faster acting than epinephrine.
    b. They prevent the release of histamines into the blood.
    c. Given before the injection of an intravenous iodinated contrast medium, they prevent an allergic reaction.
    d. They treat the symptoms of allergy but do not immunize against allergic reactions.

88. Which of the following statements is *true* concerning epinephrine?

    a. Antihistamines are faster acting than epinephrine.
    b. It prevents the release of histamines into the blood.
    c. It is usually reserved for the treatment of moderate to severe allergic reactions.
    d. It does not occur naturally in the human body.

89. If prednisone is used to premedicate a patient that is scheduled for a contrast enhanced CT examination, what is the typical method of administration?

    a. 50 mg given intravenously, just before the procedure
    b. 50 mg given intramuscularly, 1 hour before the procedure
    c. 3 doses of 50 mg given orally 13 hours, 7 hours, and 1 hour before the procedure
    d. 3 doses of 25 mg given orally 13 days, 5 days, and 3 days before the procedure

90. What property of intravenous contrast media is responsible for its capacity to increase a structure's ability to attenuate the x-ray beam?

    a. osmolality
    b. viscosity
    c. iodine concentration
    d. ionic nature

91. How does the osmolality of the newer types of contrast agents (e.g., Omnipaque®, Isovue®, Optiray®) compare with that of body fluids?

    a. They have nearly the same osmolality as body fluids.
    b. They have approximately twice the osmolality of body fluids.
    c. They have approximately five times the osmolality of body fluids.
    d. They have approximately seven times the osmolality of body fluids.

92. Which factors affect the viscosity of an intravenous iodinated contrast agent?

    1. iodine concentration
    2. lipid solubility
    3. total volume delivered
    4. temperature of the agent
        a. 1 and 2
        b. 2 and 3
        c. 1 and 4
        d. 1, 3, and 4

93. What is the approximate half-time of contrast media in patients with normal renal function?

    a. 3 minutes
    b. 30 minutes
    c. 1 to 2 hours
    d. 12 to 18 hours

94. In discussions of radiation dosimetry, for what is the quality factor used?

    a. to measure exposure in air
    b. to convert rads to centigray
    c. to measure the dose from multiple scans
    d. to account for different types of radiation

95. A CT examination of the abdomen is ordered on an 80-year-old woman. Charted laboratory values show a creatinine value of 2.7 mg/dl. Assuming the examination is performed with 150 ml of a standard 300 mgI/ml concentration of a low-osmolality contrast material, this patient has an increased risk of developing

    a. contrast medium-induced nephrotoxicity
    b. a generalized anaphylactoid reaction
    c. prominent urticaria
    d. a major convulsion or seizure

96. Why is it important to note the patient's previous oncology treatments on the history form?

    a. Some chemotherapy agents are incompatible with iodinated contrast materials.
    b. A CT examination should not be performed on the same day a radiation therapy treatment is given.
    c. Chemotherapy agents increase the patient's risk of developing contrast medium-induced acute renal failure (CM-ARF).
    d. Scarring caused by radiation therapy often mimics lung disease.

97. Which of the following concentrations provides an acceptable solution for oral contrast media used in CT?

    a. 1%–3% barium suspension or 2%–5% water-soluble solution
    b. 10%–20% solution of either barium or a water-soluble material
    c. 25% barium suspension or 10% water-soluble solution
    d. 45%–50% barium suspension or 20%–25% water-soluble solution

98. Which of the following increase the risk of bleeding following a biopsy procedure?

   1. elevated BUN and creatinine values

   2. use of a larger diameter biopsy needle

   3. highly vascularized lesion to be examined

   4. recent blood transfusion

     a. 1 and 4

     b. 1 and 2

     c. 2 and 3

     d. 1, 2, 3, and 4

99. Which of the following factors affect contrast enhancement in a CT study?

   1. the delay from start of injection to start of scanning

   2. the contrast flow rate

   3. the speed of the scanning system

   4. the iodine concentration and volume

     a. 1 and 2

     b. 1, 3, and 4

     c. 2, 3, and 4

     d. 1, 2, 3, and 4

100. The difference between the bolus, nonequilibrium, and equilibrium phases of contrast media enhancement is predominantly determined by the

   1. osmolality of the contrast

   2. rate the contrast is delivered

   3. time that has elapsed between injection and scanning

   4. the patient's size

     a. 1 and 2

     b. 2 and 3

     c. 1, 2, and 4

     d. 1, 3, and 4

101. Assuming intravenous access was unsuccessfully attempted using an 18-gauge butterfly needle set, the decision is made to switch to a smaller diameter intravenous catheter. The technologist should select which of the following equipment?

     a. 20-gauge/20 cm Chiba

     b. 20-gauge Angiocath

     c. 16-gauge Angiocath

     d. 16-gauge Franseen

102. Given *orally*, compare low-osmolality contrast medium to high-osmolality contrast medium.

     a. Low-osmolality contrast medium offers no advantage and is much more expensive.

     b. Low-osmolality contrast medium offers a clear advantage in all patients.

     c. Low-osmolality contrast media have not been approved for oral administration.

     d. In some instances, particularly with infants, low-osmolality contrast agents may provide significant advantages over the high-osmolality agents.

103. What is the appropriate way to document a charting error?

     a. Use correction fluid to eliminate the mistake, then write the correction over it.

     b. Tear out the entire sheet and insert a new one.

     c. Draw one line through the entry, and then initial, date, and enter the time at which the correction was made.

     d. Use a black marker to entirely cover the mistake and write the correction next to it.

104. Which techniques are recommended in body scanning to produce consistent and reproducible intravenous iodinated contrast enhancement?

    1. use a mechanical flow-control injector
    2. follow specified injection protocols
    3. make a notation on the patient's chart when protocols cannot be adhered to
    4. use a gravity drip infusion method
        a. 2 only
        b. 1 and 2
        c. 1, 2, and 3
        d. 1, 2, 3, and 4

105. The intravenous infusion of iodinated contrast media may result in

    a. a sharp drop in blood sugar
    b. severe fetal abnormalities if given to a pregnant woman
    c. dehydration
    d. a sensitivity to seafood

106. What are three common tests performed before a CT-guided biopsy?

    a. uric acid, BUN, serum glutamic-oxaloacetate transaminase
    b. lactate dehydrogenase, creatine phosphokinase, triglycerides
    c. partial triglyceride time, phosphatase time, bleeding time
    d. PT, partial thromboplastin timed (PTT), platelet count

107. The detector "reads" each arriving ray and measures how much of the beam has been attenuated. This is

    a. a ray sum
    b. a view
    c. back projection
    d. a sample

108. The x axis refers to

    a. the width of the pixel
    b. the height of the pixel
    c. the slice thickness
    d. the rotational nature of the x-ray tube

109. How can the total number of pixels in the matrix be calculated?

    a. multiply the number of pixels in a row by the number of pixels in a column
    b. divide the slice thickness by the display field
    c. multiply the pixel size by the display field
    d. add the number of pixels in a row to the number of pixels in a column, then multiply by the size of one pixel

110. Filling an anatomic structure with an oral or intravenous contrast agent results in

    a. an increase in the number of x-ray photons reaching the detector
    b. an increase in the structure's beam attenuation
    c. a lower radiation exposure (average absorbed dose) to the patient
    d. a decrease in pixel size

111. A structure is slightly less dense than water. What is the expected Hounsfield measurement?

    a. −970
    b. −20
    c. 30
    d. 630

112. To create x-ray, electrons are "boiled off" of a filament and then propelled across to the anode. What unit is used to refer to the amount of electrons in the stream that runs from the filament to the anode?

    a. kVp
    b. thousand heat units (KHU)
    c. mA
    d. sievert (Sv)

113. In what unit is the heat capacity of a system listed?

    a. KHU
    b. million heat units (MHU)
    c. kilowatts (kW)
    d. mAs

114. In a specific CT system, the x-ray that passes through the patient hits the detector and is converted into light. What type of detector does this system possess?

    a. solid-state
    b. xenon gas
    c. aluminum
    d. either solid-state or xenon gas

115. The reconstruction processor assigns how many Hounsfield units (HU) to each pixel in the matrix?

    a. one
    b. number of HU per pixel is one-tenth the display field of view
    c. number of HU per pixel is one-tenth the matrix size
    d. number of HU per pixel is one-tenth the display field of view divided by the matrix size

116. In a CT system, what is the function of the generator?

    a. produces an electric current of very high amperage and transmits it to the filament
    b. produces high voltage and transmits it to the x-ray tube
    c. processes thousands of bits of data per second
    d. dissipates the heat built up during x-ray production

117. Figure 4–12 illustrates a scanner with a

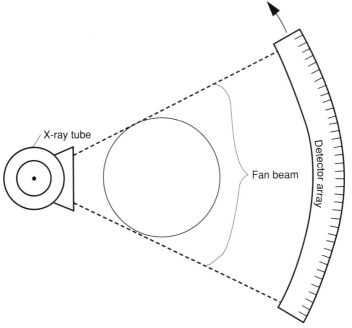

  a. second-generation design
  b. third-generation design

  c. fourth-generation design
  d. fifth-generation design

118. This type of image artifact results from lower-energy photons being preferentially absorbed, leaving higher-intensity photons to strike the detector array. This refers to

  a. sampling artifacts
  b. beam-hardening artifacts
  c. cupping artifacts
  d. photon–depravation-induced image noise

119. Reducing scatter radiation improves

  a. quantum mottle
  b. contrast resolution
  c. heat dissipation
  d. detector efficiency

120. Which qualities can be attributed to a xenon gas detector system?

  1. high detector efficiency
  2. highly stable
  3. less expensive to produce
  4. no afterglow

  a. 1 and 3
  b. 1, 2, and 3
  c. 2, 3, and 4
  d. 1, 2, 3, and 4

121. If an object is described as having a low spatial frequency, it

  a. is very dense
  b. will not be visible on a CT image
  c. will not respond to a magnetic field
  d. is relatively large

122. Concerning data acquired in a CT system, which of the following is a true statement?

    a. Image data require five times more computer storage space than raw data.
    b. Image data are often saved on auxiliary devices such as optical disks, whereas raw data are rarely archived.
    c. Most systems have computer space allotted for many more raw data files than image data files.
    d. Because of the advent of spiral scanning, manufacturers were forced to decrease the computer space allotted to raw data and increase the space allotted to image data.

123. Which of the following factors affect the pixel size?

    1. field of view
    2. detector spacing
    3. matrix size
    4. modulation transfer function (MTF)
        a. 1 and 2
        b. 2 and 4
        c. 1 and 3
        d. 1, 3, and 4

124. An exposure is made at 300 mAs and 120 kVp on both a third-generation and a fourth-generation system. Which of the following statements is true concerning radiation dose to the patient?

    a. The radiation exposure is identical.
    b. The radiation exposure is doubled with the third-generation system.
    c. The radiation exposure is higher with the fourth-generation system.
    d. The radiation exposure is entirely dependent on the type of detector used and not the scanner generation.

125. The ability of a system to define an edge is referred to as

    a. Nyquist sampling theorem
    b. receiver–operator characteristics (ROC)
    c. sharpness
    d. MTF

126. CT is superior to conventional film/screen radiography in its

    a. ability to provide radiographic images with a much lower radiation dose
    b. capacity for surveying many diverse anatomic areas quickly
    c. ability to resolve small differences in tissue densities
    d. spatial resolution

127. The subjective aspect of the quality assessment of a CT image is called

    a. ROC
    b. MTF
    c. edge response function (ERF)
    d. spatial frequency

128. A straight line radiating from a high-contrast area is determined to be an artifact caused by the edge gradient effect. What can be performed to eliminate the artifact?

    a. Calibrate or replace faulty detector.
    b. Increase kVp setting or increase filtration.
    c. Increase scan time or decrease slice thickness.
    d. Increase scan field size or increase tube cooling time.

129. Which actions reduce beam-hardening artifacts?

   a. Increase mA setting or increase scan
      time.
   b. Use a partial scan or recalibrate the
      system.
   c. Increase kVp setting or increase
      filtration.
   d. Decrease scan field size or decrease
      matrix size.

130. Which one of the following standard deviation readings indicates that a lesion is homogeneous in nature?

   a. −30
   b. 0
   c. 20
   d. 200

131. Which archival device allows the quickest re-
trieval of an image?

   a. digital audio tape (DAT)
   b. optical disk
   c. magnetic tape
   d. floppy disk

132. On a CT image a structure is measured, and
its CT number, or HU, is 0. What can be
determined about this structure?

   a. It is very homogeneous.
   b. It is very heterogeneous.
   c. It is composed of water or something
      with the same density as water.
   d. It was not large enough to obtain an
      adequate measurement.

133. In a CT image the window width is set at
300 and the level is set at 50. Which one of
the following statements is true?

   a. The liver appears gray.
   b. The linear attenuation coefficient for
      bone is 0.19 cm^{-1}.
   c. The average photon energy is 10
      kiloelectron volts (keV).
   d. The Hounsfield value of water is 50.

134. Visible fluctuations in the image that result
in a salt-and-pepper look are called

   a. quantum mottle
   b. aliasing effect
   c. image conformity
   d. nonhomogeneity

135. Increasing the kilovoltage results in an increase in the

   a. speed of the electrons as they travel
      from filament to anode
   b. number of electrons that "boil off" of
      the filament
   c. speed of electrons as they travel from
      the anode through the patient
   d. rate at which the system can rid itself of
      by-product heat

136. What is the result if too low an mAs setting
is used?

   a. The CT values, or HU, are inaccurate.
   b. The pixel size increases, corresponding
      to a decrease in spatial resolution.
   c. Vague areas of increased density in a
      somewhat concentric shape appear
      around the periphery of the image.
   d. The image has a speckled appearance
      that decreases the contrast resolution.

137. In the quality assessment of an image, a phantom with a series of narrowly spaced lines is often used. What aspect of image quality does this phantom assess?

    a. spatial resolution
    b. contrast resolution
    c. accuracy of slice thickness
    d. noise and uniformity

138. How are the electrons that make x-ray produced?

    a. High kVp is used to magnetize the target material, which then spins to produce electrons.
    b. An electric field is amplified by a photodiode, thereby producing a positively charged cloud of electrons.
    c. A wire is moved rapidly within a magnetic field, producing electrons.
    d. The filament heats up until electrons are boiled off.

139. What is an advantage of a narrow window setting?

    a. suppresses the display of image noise
    b. provides greater density discrimination between similar density objects
    c. encompasses greater anatomic diversity
    d. allows a lower mAs setting to be used

140. Which of the following are typically located within the gantry?

    1. x-ray tube
    2. detector
    3. data acquisition system (DAS)
    4. central processing unit (CPU)
        a. 1 and 2
        b. 1, 2, and 3
        c. 1, 3, and 4
        d. 1, 2, 3, and 4

141. What is the purpose of a slip-ring device in a spiral CT system?

    a. allows the table to move smoothly through the gantry
    b. improves the efficiency of the detectors
    c. allows the gantry continuous rotation
    d. increases the heat dissipation rate of the x-ray tube

142. Why might overlapping images be retrospectively created from a spiral scan series?

    a. to eliminate motion artifacts
    b. to reduce "stair-step" artifacts on a three-dimensional reformation
    c. to narrow the slice thickness
    d. to reduce the data to be archived

143. Image data can be used for

    a. changing the display field size
    b. changing the reconstruction algorithm
    c. creating a multiplanar reformation
    d. creating overlapping images from spiral data

144. Keeping all other factors constant, increasing the pitch from 1 to 2 (1:1 to 2:1) results in

    a. more anatomy being covered
    b. increased tube heat
    c. improved spatial resolution in the z axis
    d. increased total examination time

145. Which is a disadvantage inherent in producing images with good low-contrast resolution?

    a. higher radiation dose
    b. poor spatial resolution
    c. small images
    d. use of a wide gray scale

146. Periodically testing the performance of a CT scanner and comparing its performance with an established standard is

a. required daily by federal law
b. a quality control program
c. not necessary because quality control programs are built into all CT scanners
d. performed exclusively by the service engineers

147. Which of the following statements is true concerning multiplanar reformation?

a. In general, the thinner the original slice, the better the reformatted image.
b. Using overlapping images degrades the reformation.
c. Spiral data cannot be used for sagittal reformations.
d. Reformatted images are of equal or better quality than actually scanning in another plane.

148. In Figure 4–13, what is the object marked X called?

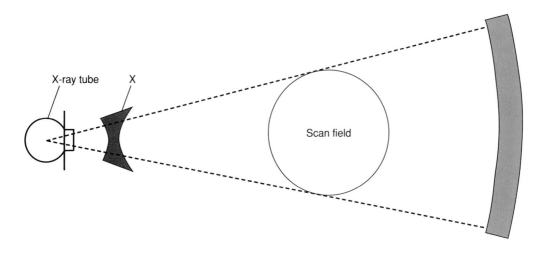

a. collimator
b. bow tie filter

c. focal spot
d. reference detector

149. In a third-generation design system, where are the reference detectors usually located?

a. at either end of the detector array
b. between each of the regular detectors in the array
c. near the collimator
d. in the CPU

150. What is an attenuation profile?

a. the process of converting all the acquired data to a matrix
b. the result of accounting for the attenuation properties of each ray sum and correlating them with the position of the ray
c. the result of applying a filter function to data
d. the computer file created for each image, so that it can be archived

Answers and Explanations

1. **Answer-d.** Cerebral infarctions are often called strokes. They are caused by a blockage of the blood supply to a region of the brain, which results in necrosis or cystic change. Because there is no blood supply to the region, infarcts do not respond to contrast enhancement.

2. **Answer-c**

3. **Answer-c**

4. **Answer-b**

5. **Answer-b.** Because volume averaging, or partial volume effect, is reduced when slice thickness is reduced, the likelihood of detecting small lesions increases.

6. **Answer-d.** Exceptions to the rule are lesions located in areas without an intact blood–brain barrier, such as the pituitary gland or cavernous sinuses. In these situations, a bolus injection followed by rapid sequence scanning is effective.

7. **Answer-a.** The arachnoid membrane encloses the brain and spinal cord and is separated from the pia mater (inner membrane) by the subarachnoid space. The dura mater is the outer membrane and is separated from the arachnoid membrane by the subdural space.

8. **Answer-a.** Images created using a high-contrast algorithm are particularly useful in evaluating bony deterioration of the small structures of the inner ear.

9. **Answer-d.** The small, complicated structures of the osteomeatal complex are best visualized with a thin slice.

10. **Answer-a.** Hyperextension of the neck should be avoided because it may obstruct the patient's airway in those patients with a neck mass. Choices c and d are used to evaluate the aryepiglottic folds and pyriform sinuses. Spiral scanning is often used in neck scanning to allow all scans to be acquired when the patient suspends swallowing.

11. **Answer-c.** Because the thorax has the highest intrinsic natural contrast of any body part, many radiologists feel that additional contrast enhancement is not routinely needed. Because spiral scanning is accomplished so quickly, it is necessary to allow the contrast medium enough time to circulate. A biphasic injection is of value when an older, slower scanning system is used.

12. **Answer-a**

13. **Answer-d**

14. **Answer-c.** Overlapping slices improve reformations by reducing the "stair-step" appearance common in reformatted images. Other factors that can improve a multiplanar reformation are scanning with a thin slice and reducing or eliminating motion. Using a short scan time helps to reduce motion artifacts.

15. **Answer-a.** Radiologists often compare an unenhanced image to its enhanced counterpart to characterize an abnormality by evaluating its enhancement pattern. These comparisons are more easily made when enhanced and unenhanced slices are taken at identical table positions.

16. **Answer-d.** The glabellomeatal line is approximately 15° cephalad to the orbital meatal line. By setting the slice angle at the acanthomeatal line, the lens of the eye, which is somewhat sensitive to radiation, receives less exposure.

17. **Answer-d**

18. **Answer-b**

19. **Answer-a**

20. **Answer-b**

21. **Answer-d.** This technique is used to improve spatial resolution by reducing the pixel size. High-resolution computed tomography (CT) is typically performed with a thin slice taken at large intervals, without intravenous contrast media.

22. **Answer-c.** Because all scans can be completed before the equilibrium phase, precontrasted studies of the liver are often eliminated. Research has shown that contrast dose may be reduced by as much as 33% when a spiral technique is used to replace an older, slower system. A mechanical flow-control injector becomes even more important as contrast timing is more critical with a fast scan technique. Total scan time is reduced when using a fast scanner; therefore, an increased patient throughput can be expected.

23. **Answer-a.** The adrenal glands are by far the most common location for pheochromocytomas. The next most common location is the organ of Zuckerkandl, which is just below the aortic bifurcation.

24. **Answer-a.** "Fatty infiltration of the liver is the result of excessive deposition of triglyceride which occurs in association with a variety of disorder including obesity, malnutrition, chemotherapy hyperalimentation, alcohol abuse, steroid administration, Cushing's syndrome and radiation hepatitis."[1]

25. **Answer-c.** The pons also contains the centers for reflexes, which are mediated by the fifth, sixth, seventh, and eighth cranial nerves. The pons also regulates respiration.

26. **Answer-c.** The dynamic range of a detector used in a CT system is up to 10,000 to 1, compared with approximately 100 to 1 in film/screen radiography.

27. **Answer-d.** Because of the increased collimation, a narrower slice results in fewer x-ray photons. To compensate, milliampere-seconds (mAs) must be increased.

28. **Answer-c.** In this spiral scan technique, the tube requires 1 second to make a complete rotation; with no other changes, the resulting mAs would be 150. Spiral scans require approximately the same total mAs as those taken in an axial method; therefore, milliamperes (mA) must be increased to compensate for the shortened scan time.

29. **Answer-c**

30. **Answer-d**

31. **Answer-c.** The sphenoid bone constitutes the center portion of the cranial floor and forms part of the orbit's floor and sidewalls.

[1] Baron R, Freeny P, Moss A: Abdomen and pelvis. In *Computed Tomography of the Body, with Magnetic Resonance Imaging,* 2nd ed, vol. 3. Edited by Moss A. Philadelphia, WB Saunders, 1992, p 751.

32. Answer-b. The pituitary gland is actually two glands: the anterior pituitary, or the adenohypophysis, and the posterior pituitary, or the neurohypophysis.

33. Answer-d. The anatomy of a spiral scan acquisition can be determined by the following formula

Total acquisition time

$$\times \frac{1}{\text{Rotation time}} \times \text{Slice thickness}$$

$$\times \text{ Pitch}$$

$$= \text{Amount of anatomy covered}$$

Therefore, using the original parameters

20-second acquisition time

$$\times \frac{1}{\text{1-second rotation time}}$$

$$\times \text{ 7-mm slice thickness}$$

$$\times \text{ 1 pitch} = \text{140-mm anatomy covered}$$

This shows that we are 60 mm too short, so the new parameter should cover 200 mm of anatomy (140 mm + 60).

Choice 1:

$$20 \text{ seconds} \times \frac{1}{1} \times 10 \text{ mm} \times 1 = 200 \text{ mm}$$

Choice 2:

$$20 \text{ seconds} \times \frac{1}{1} \times 7 \text{ mm} \times 1.5 = 210 \text{ mm}$$

Choice 3:

$$20 \text{ seconds} \times \frac{1}{1.5} \times 7 \text{ mm} \times 1 = 93 \text{ mm}$$

Choice 4:

$$29 \text{ seconds} \times \frac{1}{1} \times 7 \text{ mm} \times 1 = 203 \text{ mm}$$

Choices 1, 2, and 4 succeed in covering the area of interest. The choice selected would be largely dependent on how the individual system handles tube heat loading. Choices 1 and 2 would not increase the heat loading.

34. Answer-c. In addition to the fact that CT images provide precise localization of lesions, CT images permit the clinician to plan an access route to the lesion by showing its relation with surrounding structures. Procedures can be performed on small lesions because the tip of the needle within the structure can be seen. Another advantage is that patients can be placed in a variety of positions to allow easier access to the lesion.

35. Answer-b

36. Answer-a

37. Answer-c

38. Answer-d

39. Answer-d

40. Answer-b. Overlapping slices occur in conventional axial CT studies when slice spacing is less than slice thickness. A common example is in lumbar spine studies where the slice thickness is 5 mm and the slice spacing is either 3 or 4 mm. Overlapping slices increase the radiation exposure to the patient and have no effect on beam hardening.

41. Answer-c. Lipomas are fatty tumors that are very often multiple but are not metastatic.

42. Answer-a. What are typically referred to as "lung windows" are settings with a wide window width to encompass the density diversity, and a center near the average density of lung tissue.

43. Answer-b

44. Answer-a

45. Answer-a

46. **Answer-a**

47. **Answer-b**

48. **Answer-b**

49. **Answer-c**

50. **Answer-b**

51. **Answer-a**

52. **Answer-b**

53. **Answer-d.** If the scan data were acquired in a spiral mode, it is possible to create overlapping slices by changing the incrementation of data. This may allow a lesion that straddled two slices in the initial images to fall completely within a single slice. This results in less data from normal tissue being averaged in with the lesion's data. See Figure 4–14.

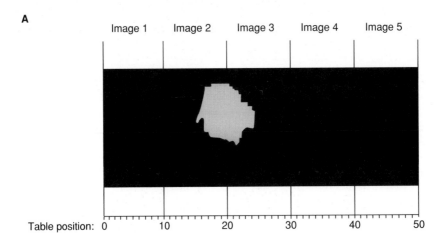

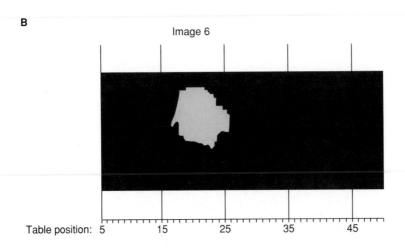

54. **Answer-d**

55. **Answer-a**

56. **Answer-b**

57. **Answer-d**

58. **Answer-a**

59. **Answer-a**

60. **Answer-a**

61. **Answer-b**

62. **Answer-a**

63. **Answer-c**

64. **Answer-d**

65. **Answer-a**

66. **Answer-c.** Bone windows also help to visualize any bony destruction resulting from intracranial lesions.

67. **Answer-c.** All stereotactic systems require the purchase of a localizing device. This hardware is placed on the CT scanning table.

68. **Answer-b**

69. **Answer-d**

70. **Answer-a**

71. **Answer-d.** The word sinus has been given to two entirely different kinds of spaces connected with the skull. Sinuses external to the cranium are hollow spaces, such as the ethmoid and sphenoid paranasal sinuses. Sinuses in the interior of the cranium, which produce grooves on the inner surface of the bones, are venous channels along which the blood runs in its passage back from the brain.

72. **Answer-c.** The three vessels arising from the aortic arch are the brachiocephalic artery, the left common carotid artery, and the left subclavian artery, respectively.

73. **Answer-c**

74. **Answer-d**

75. **Answer-a**

76. **Answer-b**

77. **Answer-d.** Choice a is the definition of antibody, b describes the term infarct, and c is characteristic of a thrombus.

78. **Answer-c.** Viscosity or "thickness" of the medium is an important physical property that influences the injectability or delivery through small-bore needles and intravenous catheters. When temperature is increased from room to body temperature, the viscosity of a contrast medium solution decreases.

79. **Answer-b.** Reactions are classified into four groups: minor, moderate, major, and fatal. Moderate reactions are usually not life threatening but require some treatment.

80. **Answer-b.** The normal range is 10 to 15 seconds.

81. **Answer-d.** The purpose of skin preparation is to minimize the introduction of pathogens into the body via the puncture or incision, thus reducing the likelihood of infection. Hair removal is not always required for skin preparation, and shaving is performed only on the specific order of the physician in charge.

82. **Answer-b.** An individual that is very athletic has a lower heart rate because his heart has been conditioned to work more efficiently.

83. **Answer-c.** The carotid artery is readily accessible and is particularly important if a patient loses consciousness. If the pulse is not discernible at this site, emergency measures are necessary.

84. **Answer-a.** Patients suffering from shock or a significant blood loss have a marked increase in pulse rate and exhibit rapid, shallow breathing. This is a result of the body's attempt to supply oxygen to the tissues by increasing the circulatory speed.

85. **Answer-b.** The average blood pressure in a healthy adult is generally considered to be approximately 120/80. A diastolic pressure of less than 50 mm Hg may indicate shock, whereas greater than 90 mm Hg indicates some degree of hypertension.

86. **Answer-a.** There are several other general housekeeping rules as well: always clean from top down, avoid raising dust, do not contaminate yourself or clean areas, every piece of equipment that comes in contact with the patient must be cleaned after each use, and only cleaning agents specified by hospital policies should be used.

87. **Answer-d.** In an allergic reaction, histamines are released into the blood. Histamine response can be opposed by two types of drugs, the rapidly acting epinephrine and the more slowly acting group of antihistamines. Antihistamines can reduce the severity of the symptoms observed in the allergic patient but do not prevent histamine release. Therefore, they treat only the symptoms of allergy and do not immunize the patient against allergic reactions. Antihistamines are more effective if taken when symptoms first appear.

88. **Answer-c.** Epinephrine is in a class of drugs called adrenergic agents. They occur naturally in the human body, with epinephrine primarily secreted from the adrenal medulla. It can be synthetically manufactured and may be administered to produce the same effects as its naturally secreted counterpart. Epinephrine is much faster acting than antihistamines and consequently is used to treat more severe allergic reactions.

89. **Answer-c.** Although many different schedules exist for premedicating a patient with prednisone, all require the oral administration of 50 mg prednisone beginning from 3 days to 13 hours before the procedure. A second dose is given from 24 to 7 hours before the examination. The third and final dose is most often given 1 hour before the procedure, but alternately may be given immediately following examination completion. In addition to the prednisone, diphenhydramine hydrochloride (Benadryl) is sometimes given 1 hour before the examination. Premedication of patients reduces but does not eliminate anaphylactoid-type reactions.

90. **Answer-c.** The iodine atoms in the contrast material are exclusively responsible for an enhanced structure's increased beam attenuation capacity. The degree to which this occurs is directly related to the concentration of iodine in the contrast material.

91. **Answer-b.** The newer, or low-osmolality, contrast agents have approximately twice the osmolality of blood. Although an osmolality that matches body fluids is the ideal, newer agents offer a great improvement over

the older agents, which have up to seven times the osmolality of blood. This decrease in osmolality is why fewer side effects are experienced with the use of the low-osmolality agents.

92. **Answer-c.** Viscosity can be described as the thickness or friction of the fluid as it flows. In the case of intravenous iodinated contrast agents, a higher concentration of iodine results in a more viscous solution. Heating the agents from room temperature to body temperature significantly decreases the solution's viscosity.

93. **Answer-c.** Renal clearance is typically described by the term half-time, which is the time required for one half of the iodine to be cleared. In patients with normal renal function, the half-time is between 1 and 2 hours for all classes of contrast agents.

94. **Answer-d.** In recognition of the health effects of x-ray, a conversion factor called the quality factor is applied to the absorbed dose. This accounts for the different health effects produced from varing types of ionizing radiations. This value is for the diagnostic x-rays that are used in CT. The quality factor is usually written as a Q.

95. **Answer-a.** A creatinine level of over 2.0 mg/dl may indicate preexisting renal insufficiency. This is a condition that places the patient at an increased risk for developing contrast medium-induced acute renal failure (CM-ARF). Careful patient screening before the injection of contrast medium reduces the incidence of CM-ARF.

96. **Answer-d.** An accurate patient history is helpful for the radiologist, particularly when evaluating changes in the lung.

97. **Answer-a.** Dilute solutions of barium sulfate and water-soluble contrast material are used for bowel opacification in CT. Either type of oral contrast produces comparable results. Because of the low concentrations used, neither coats the mucosa significantly but simply fills the bowel.

98. **Answer-c.** The primary complication of biopsy procedures is bleeding. Blood urea nitrogen (BUN) and creatinine levels indicate renal function, not a bleeding disorder. Abnormal laboratory values of prothrombin time (PT), partial thromboplastin time (PTT), and platelet count would indicate a problem.

99. **Answer-d.** The factors within a technologist's control are referred to as pharmacokinetic factors. They are iodine concentration, contrast media volume, flow rate, flow duration, scan delay time, and the total scan time.

100. **Answer-b.** The bolus phase immediately follows an intravenous bolus injection. The nonequilibrium phase follows the bolus phase. The latter most phase is the equilibrium phase, which occurs approximately 2.5 to 3 minutes after the bolus phase or following drip infusion. It is accepted that the equilibrium phase is the worst stage, particularly for hepatic scanning.

101. **Answer-b.** The gauge indicates the diameter of the needle. As the gauge increases, the diameter of the bore decreases. Neither Chiba nor Franseen needles are appropriate for venipuncture; they are typically used in biopsy procedures.

102. **Answer-d.** Research with pediatric patients has concluded that low-osmolality contrast medium offers a significant reduction in complications compared with either barium sulfate or hyperosmolar water-soluble substances. Low-osmolality contrast agents are

indicated when the possibility of entry of the contrast agent into the lung exists or when the possibility of leakage of contrast agent from the gastrointestinal tract exists. Refer to product literature for dilution protocols.

103. **Answer-c.** This method of correcting a charting error has the lowest potential for being misinterpreted if the document is reviewed later for possible litigation.

104. **Answer-c.** Using the gravity drip infusion method of contrast enhancement, the flow rate varies between studies, dependent on many factors. Some of the possible variables are the height of the bottle, the intravenous catheter size, and the viscosity of the contrast medium. Flow-control injectors are recommended to consistently produce the same level of enhancement. In addition, scanning protocols must be developed by each facility and adhered to religiously. Any deviations from set protocols must be documented so that follow-up studies of the same patient provide similar enhancement.

105. **Answer-c.** Dehydration may result from contrast media administration because the difference in osmolality between the agent and body fluids causes a shift of fluids from the cellular spaces into the plasma.

106. **Answer-d.** These laboratory tests are performed to identify a bleeding disorder, which is a contraindication for percutaneous biopsy.

107. **Answer-a.** The path the x-ray beam takes from the tube to the detector is referred to as a ray. After the ray reaches the detector and its attenuation accounted for, it is called a ray sum.

108. **Answer-a.** A pixel, or square of data, has two dimensions, width and height. Width is often referred to as the x axis, whereas the height is the y axis.

109. **Answer-a.** The total number of pixels is the number of pixels across times the number down. In a 512 matrix the total would be 512×512 or 262,144.

110. **Answer-b.** Oral or intravenous administration of a contrast agent fills the structure with a higher-density material, which increases the structure's beam attenuation.

111. **Answer-b.** In the Hounsfield system, the attenuation capacity of water is assigned 0, that of air -1000, and that of bone 1000. Objects with a beam attenuation less than that of water have an associated negative number. If an object is slightly less dense than water, a Hounsfield unit (HU) of slightly less than 0 can be expected.

112. **Answer-c.** The quantity of electrons propelled is typically referred to as tube current and is measured in one thousandth of an ampere, or 1 milliampere.

113. **Answer-b**

114. **Answer-a.** Solid-state systems are often referred to as scintillators because they emit a brief flash of light when struck by x-ray.

115. **Answer-a.** Regardless of any other factors, 1 HU is assigned to each pixel in the image matrix. This value represents the average of all density measurements for that pixel.

116. **Answer-b.** The generator produces high voltage [kilovolt (kV)] and transmits it to the x-ray tube. This high voltage propels the electrons from the x-ray tube filament to the anode. High amperage is not necessary for the production of x-ray.

117. **Answer-b.** In the third-generation design both the tube and detector array move in a circular path within the gantry. Second-generation scanners are no longer used. Electron

beam imaging is occasionally referred to as the fifth generation of CT scanning. It utilizes a large electron gun as its x-ray source and is significantly different from other CT designs.

118. **Answer-b.** Because x-ray is comprised of photons of varying intensities, the "softer" beams are more readily absorbed, leaving only the "harder" beams to reach the detector.

119. **Answer-b.** Reducing scatter radiation improves contrast resolution, which is the ability to differentiate small density differences on the image. Reducing scatter also lowers the radiation dose to the patient.

120. **Answer-c.** Because xenon gas must be kept under pressure in aluminum casings, some of the x-ray is absorbed by the casing and does not reach the detector. This loss in the detector window is the main reason that efficiency is hampered in a xenon gas system. As a result, the efficiency of a xenon gas detector is significantly lower than a solid-state system.

121. **Answer-d.** How frequently an object will fit into a given space will determine spatial frequency. Therefore, large objects have low spatial frequency, and small objects have high spatial frequency.

122. **Answer-b.** In most cases, raw data cannot be saved on an auxiliary device. Because raw data include all measurements obtained from the detector array, it requires approximately five times the computer space as image data. Most CT systems have 4 to 10 times more image files than raw data files. In spiral scanning, the data are obtained much faster than the computer can process the data into images. The raw data must be stored while awaiting reconstruction. For this reason, raw data storage is expanded for spiral scanning.

123. **Answer-c.** The display field of view and the matrix determine pixel size. The formula is: Pixel size = field of view divided by matrix size.

124. **Answer-c.** All other factors remaining constant, the exposure is higher in the fourth-generation system in which the tube is closer to the patient because the tube rotates within the ring of detectors. This follows the inverse square law.

125. **Answer-c.** Sharpness is the ability of a system to define an edge. It is measured by the amount of blur in a system.

126. **Answer-c.** The ability to distinguish objects with similar densities is called low-contrast resolution. CT images have lower spatial resolution and much higher low-contrast discrimination than that of conventional film/screen radiography.

127. **Answer-a.** Two viewers may evaluate the same image differently, thereby coming to somewhat different conclusions. To illustrate, image quality is commonly evaluated by using a line pair (lp) phantom such as the one in Figure 4–15. One observer may view Figure 4–15 and clearly identify 15 lp (an lp is one line and one space), whereas a second observer may feel only 12 lp per centimeter are clearly visible. This subjectivity is referred to as receiver–operator characteristics (ROC).

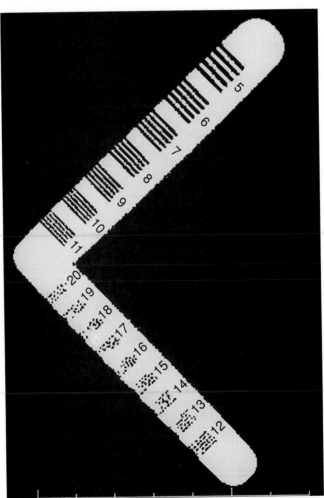

Figure 4-15. The line pair phantom is used to evaluate spatial resolution.

128. **Answer-c.** Edge gradient effect artifacts are created when the angle of the x-ray beam varies between two similar views. This can be reduced or eliminated by increasing the scan time or decreasing the slice thickness.

129. **Answer-c.** Beam-hardening artifacts result from the fact that the x-ray beam is polychromatic. Therefore, any action that reduces the range of x-ray beam energies also reduces these artifacts. Increasing the kilovolt-peak (kVp) increases the average photon energy, and increasing the filtration removes many of the lower-energy, or "soft," photons.

130. **Answer-b.** The standard deviation indicates the variation of pixel values within a given region of interest. If there is a wide variety of pixel readings, the standard deviation is high. If every pixel within the region has the same value, the standard deviation is zero. The standard deviation cannot be a negative number; it is always greater than or equal to zero.

131. **Answer-b.** Although optical disks are typically the most expensive option for data storage, they allow the quickest access to data.

132. **Answer-c.** On the Hounsfield scale, water is assigned the number 0, so the structure must be water or some other material with the same density. It is not possible to tell from the Hounsfield measurement alone whether the structure is homogeneous. The standard deviation reading would help to evaluate that aspect of the structure.

133. **Answer-a.** Because the Hounsfield value of liver tissue falls near the middle of the display range, it is represented by a shade of gray. Neither the linear attenuation coefficient nor the average photon energy can be determined with the information given. Window settings do not change Hounsfield values, only their appearance on the image.

134. **Answer-a.** Quantum mottle is also referred to as image noise. It results from an insufficient number of photons reaching the detectors and reduces the contrast resolution in an image.

135. **Answer-a.** Electrons "boil off" of the heated filament and are propelled across to strike the anode, where they disarrange the target material to produce x-ray. The x-ray photons (not electrons) then travel from the anode to the patient. Increasing the kilovoltage increases the speed in which they travel. Ultimately, this results in a higher photon energy of the resultant x-ray.

136. **Answer-d.** The mAs setting determines how much x-ray is produced. Too low a setting results in an insufficient amount of x-ray photons reaching the detectors. This causes a speckled appearance on the image, which is typically referred to as noise or quantum mottle. Image noise makes it more difficult to differentiate objects with similar densities.

137. **Answer-a.** Spatial resolution is often reported as the number of line pairs visible. A line pair is *not* defined as a set of two lines, rather it is considered a line and the adjacent space. It is typically abbreviated as lp/cm.

138. **Answer-d.** To produce electrons, a filament is heated until electrons are emitted to form a negatively charged cloud around the filament. This cloud is called a space charge.

139. **Answer-b.** Narrow window widths are typically used when tissue densities are similar, such as the gray and white matter of the brain. A rule of thumb to enhance contrast between two tissues is: narrow the window to just include both and set the level centered between them.

140. Answer-b. The gantry houses imaging components including the x-ray tube, detectors, data acquisition system (sometimes called detector electronics), collimators, slip rings, and a high-tension generator. The central processing unit (CPU) is not located within the gantry but may be near the operator's console or in a separate computer room.

141. Answer-c. The use of a slip-ring device in a CT system eliminates long, high-tension cables that have to be unwound after each rotation. This allows the tube to rotate in a single direction rather than stopping after each 360° rotation to turn in the opposing direction.

142. Answer-b. Overlapping images create a smoother reformatted image. An advantage to spiral scanning is that because these overlapping images are performed by reconstructing the data set, they do not increase radiation exposure to the patient as in conventional CT.

143. Answer-c. Multiplanar reformation software stack up images, and then slice the stacked whole body part in a plane specified by the operator. These can be created from image data, providing the images possess the same display field size, center, and gantry tilt; and the slices are contiguous.

144. Answer-a. Doubling the pitch increases the table speed so that twice as much anatomy is covered during one tube rotation.

145. Answer-a. The radiation dose for CT examinations is substantially higher than those for film/screen studies of the same body part. This higher dose is required to suppress quantum noise and provide the good low-contrast resolution that is the hallmark of CT images.

146. Answer-b. A consistent quality control program is recommended by all CT manufacturers to ensure a system is operating at peak efficiency. Federal law does not regulate the specifics of a quality control program. It is left to the individual facility to design a program that is appropriate for their site.

147. Answer-a. Overlapping slices are often used to reduce the "stair-step" look of a reformatted image. Spiral scans are particularly good for reformation because slices can be retrospectively reconstructed to produce overlapping images without exposing the patient to an increased radiation dose. Although image reformatting is useful and often provides additional information, the images produced are not comparable with those actually scanned in another plane.

148. Answer-b. Mechanical filters shape the x-ray beam intensity. Filtering removes soft, or low-energy, x-ray beams and minimizes patient exposure. Bow tie filters are used to reduce the beam intensity at the periphery of the beam, corresponding to the thinner areas of a patient's anatomy.

149. Answer-a. Reference detectors are located at the ends of the detector array and measure only the unattenuated x-ray beam.

150. Answer-b. An attenuation profile is created for each view in the scan. Applying a filter function is called convolution.

Suggested Reading

Physics

Behrman R: *Study Guide to Computed Tomography*, vols. 1 and 2. Greenwich, CT, Clinical Communication Inc., 1995.

Berland L: *Practical CT: Technology and Techniques*. New York, Raven Press, 1987.

Bushong S: *Radiologic Science for Technologists*. Chicago, CV Mosby, 1993.

Fishman E, Jeffrey R: *Spiral CT: Principles, Techniques, and Clinical Applications*. New York, Raven Press, 1995.

Romans L: *Introduction to Computed Tomography*. Baltimore, Williams & Wilkins, 1995.

Seeram E: *Computed Tomography: Physical Prinicples, Clinical Applications & Quality Control*. Philadelphia, WB Saunders, 1994.

Advanced Patient Care

Clayton B, Stock Y: *Basic Pharmacology for Nurses*. Chicago, CV Mosby, 1989.

Duddy M, Manns A, Wormald S: Injection rate: A factor in contrast reactions? *Clin Radiol* Volume 41, 42–43, 1990.

Dufalla T: *Intravenous Contrast Administration for Optimal Results*. Pittsburgh, Medrad, Inc., 1994.

Ehrlich R, McCloskey E: *Patient Care in Radiography*. Chicago, CV Mosby, 1993.

Greenberger P, Patterson R, Tapio C: Prophylaxis against repeated radiocontrast media reactions in 857 cases. *Arch Intern Med* 145:2197–2200, 1985.

Huda W, Stone R: *Review of Radiologic Physics*. Baltimore, Williams & Wilkins, 1995, p 135.

Joint Advisory Notice: Department of Labor/Department of Health and Human Serves; HBV/HIV: Protection against occupational exposure to hepatitis B virus and human immunodeficiency virus. *General Register* 52(Oct 30):41818–41824, 1987.

Katzberg R: *The Contrast Media Manual*. Baltimore, Williams & Wilkins, 1992.

Langer R, Kaufman HJ: The use of nonionic contrast medium for gastrointestinal studies in infants. Presented at the 72nd Scientific Assembly and Annual meeting of the RSNA, Chicago, November 30 to December 6, 1986.

Luckman J, Sorensen K: *Medical-Surgical Nursing*. Philadelphia, WB Saunders, 1980.

Mallinckrodt Medical, Inc.: *Handbook of Computed Tomography: Techniques & Protocols*. St. Louis, Mallinckrodt Medical, Inc., 1992.

Rambo B, Wood L: *Nursing Skills for Clinical Practice*. Philadelphia, WB Saunders, 1980.

Romans L: *Introduction to Computed Tomography*. Baltimore, Williams & Wilkins, 1995.

Imaging Procedures

Anthony C, Kolthoff N: *Textbook of Anatomy and Physiology*. Chicago, CV Mosby, 1975.

Chiu L, Lipcamom J, Yiu-Chiu V: *Clinical Computed Tomography for the Technologist*. New York, Raven Press, 1995.

Fishman E, Jeffrey R: *Spiral CT: Principles, Techniques, and Clinical Applications.* New York, Raven Press, 1995.

Gray H: *Gray's Anatomy.* Philadelphia, Running Press, 1974.

Hasso A, Shakudo M: *Pocket Atlas of Normal CT Anatomy of the Head and Brain.* New York, Raven Press, 1990.

Möller T, Reif E: *Pocket Atlas of Cross-Sectional Anatomy CT and MRI.* Vol. 1: Head, neck, spine, and joints. New York, Thieme, 1994.

Möller T, Reif E: *Pocket Atlas of Cross-Sectional Anatomy CT and MRI.* Vol. 2: Thorax, abdomen, and pelvis. New York, Thieme, 1994.

Novelline R, Squire L: *Living Anatomy.* Chicago, CV Mosby, 1987.

Romans L: *Introduction to Computed Tomography.* Baltimore, Williams & Wilkins, 1995.

Silverman P, Fishman E: *Helical CT: The New Standard in Computed Tomography.* Washington, DC, Georgetown University Medical Center, 1995.

Thomas C: *Taber's Cyclopedic Medical Dictionary.* Philadelphia, FA Davis, 1989.

Weinstein J, Lee J, Sagel S: *Pocket Atlas of Normal CT Anatomy.* New York, Raven Press, 1985.

Zeman R: CT angiography: Practical approaches, techniques and protocols. *Helical (Spiral) CT Today.* 1: Spring, 1995.